Adult Aural Rehabilitation

MARYANNE TATE MALTBY
DASED, BA, MEd, MSc, EdD, Dip Psych.
Senior Lecturer and Audiology Pathway Leader
Anglia Ruskin University, Cambridge.

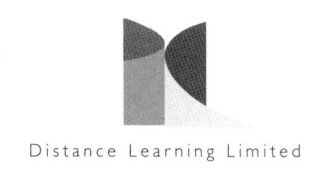

Distance Learning Limited

© First Edition published 2009 by Distance Learning Ltd
Distance Learning Ltd
La Villiaze
St Andrews
Guernsey
GY6 8YP

All rights reserved. No part of this publication may be reproduced, stored in a retrieval system, or transmitted in any form or by any means, electronic, mechanical, photocopying, recording or otherwise, without the prior permission of Distance Learning Ltd.

This publication is sold subject to the conditions that it shall not, by way of trade or otherwise, be lent, resold, hired out, or otherwise circulated without the publisher's prior consent in any form of binding or cover other than in which it is published and without a similar condition including this condition being imposed upon any subsequent purchaser.

ISBN 978-0-9563180-0-8

Contents

Preface		vii
Acknowledgements		ix
1	Introduction	1
2	The Impact of Hearing Loss	13
3	The Ageing Process	36
4	Beginning the Rehabilitation Process	61
5	Amplification	77
6	A Psychosocial Framework	99
7	Communication and Auditory Training	120
8	Counselling	149
9	Anxiety, Depression and Therapy	166
10	Evaluation	182
11	Assistive Devices	195
12	Tinnitus	214
13	Pre-Lingual Deafness	232
Appendix		251
Bibliography		255
References		267
Index		283

Preface

The sense of hearing allows us to detect the faintest of sounds in the environment and at the other extreme to be able to tolerate the loudest sounds. In between these limits it allows us to communicate effectively even in noisy backgrounds. This ability to communicate with ease is taken for granted by all of us. The problems and difficulties we may face in the absence or reduction in hearing are not given any thought. Indeed it is difficult to imagine and not easy to create a scenario where loss of hearing and its effects on the individual may be experienced.

Even for those who train to be audiologists or practise as audiologists, it is not easy to appreciate the extent of the impact of hearing impairment on the quality of life of those affected. Depending on the age at which the loss of hearing occurs, communication difficulties can result in a significant effect on education, employment and social relationships.

This book provides a much needed introduction to the processes and consequences of the loss of hearing. The impact of a hearing loss on the individual, their family and social life are described in a simple, clear and lucid style.

It will be valuable for all the people whose lives are affected by loss of hearing as well as those who are in close contact with the people affected such as family or friends and indeed the audiologists who must provide the necessary guidance and care for a successful rehabilitation programme. It leads the audiologists through a structured approach to rehabilitation explaining each step in a way that can only have come from a great deal of experience.

The practical approach to the whole process of rehabilitation from hearing aid provision, through counselling and coping strategies is covered in a well structured manner whilst providing in-depth advice at each level. The importance of the psychological and sociological aspects of rehabilitation processes cannot be emphasised enough for the audiologist.

What is unique in this book is the way the book handles the patient's as well as the audiologist's perspective so that each may understand the other's point of view of a given process in the rehabilitation programme which will lead to effective restoration in communication after the loss.

Deepak Prasher
Emeritus Professor of Audiology (University College London)
Currently Head of Audiology Department at the Royal Surrey County Hospital
Guildford
February 2009

Acknowledgements

I would like to thank all those colleagues who provided encouragement, material and suggestions, or who read the draft chapters and provided helpful comments. In particular, I wish to thank David Baguley (Addenbrookes Hospital), John Popplestone and David Evans (Connevans), Gill Robinson and Katie Trapp (Distance Learning Ltd), Kerry Tate (Islington Primary Care Trust), David Rist (Hidden Hearing), Lee Dean and Julie Chammings (Specsavers), Christine de Placido (St Margarets University, Edinburgh), Helen Belcher (Oticon) and David Gaszczyk (Self-employed audiologist). In addition I would like to thank all those companies who were so helpful in providing photographs and other materials, these included Phonak, Starkey, Pure Tone, PCWerth and Connevans. If I have forgotten anyone, I hope they will forgive me. Then finally I would like to thank Frances and her brother for permission to use her photographs.

Chapter 1
Introduction

1.1 COMMUNICATION DIFFICULTY

1.1.1 Hearing loss

Hearing is basic to human communication. Hearing loss impairs communication which in turn affects the individual, their family, friends and colleagues. The situation can be stressful for everyone.

Even a relatively mild hearing loss may cause communication difficulty. The degree of difficulty is not only dependent on the degree of hearing loss but, to a great extent, it is dependent on the individual's lifestyle. Employment, family and social life may all be greatly affected. Nevertheless, many people are unwilling to accept that they have a hearing loss at all, or at least that they may have need of hearing aids. The impact of hearing loss is explored in Chapter 2.

Hearing aids can minimise communication difficulties but appropriate fitting of hearing aids is not the end of the process. The hearing impaired individual, and those who communicate most with them, will also benefit from advice, support and counselling.

1.1.2 Managing hearing loss – the change process

Changes are inevitable in life but changes also cause us emotional upheaval. A hearing loss causes a change that seems to move the person away from 'normality'. Such a change causes anxiety and is difficult to deal with socially and emotionally. Chapter 6 introduces change management and the change transition curve in relation to hearing loss. The individual is likely to need help in coming to manage the change successfully. Rehabilitation is the journey through which the audiologist will support a client in taking the steps needed to reach a positive outcome.

Every change signals the end of something that was there before. Hearing loss signals the end of normal hearing. The future can seem uncertain and feelings of confusion and fear will usually have to be overcome before the client can move forward. The client needs time to accept, understand and express the various emotions that accompany life changes and help to take the steps that will assist them to move on.

Of course, not everyone goes through exactly the same emotions but there are certain emotional stages that are common in any change process, often starting with denial. Many people deny that they have a hearing loss and when they are forced to accept it they may experience emotions such as anger, sorrow, stress, withdrawal, etc. Once the hearing loss has been accepted, a solution can be sought and the client may go through a period of euphoria during which they think they can regain normal hearing. This period has to be managed carefully because unrealistic expectations lead to disappointment and a period of difficulty, disenchantment and depression that is sometimes referred to as the 'pit'. The support of the audiologist can help the client to focus on realistic objectives and to develop the coping skills and confidence they need to climb out of the pit and achieve their objectives.

1.1.3 Stigma

Deafness is an 'invisible' condition and many hearing impaired individuals deny even having hearing problems and, if they wear them, they want their hearing aids to be inconspicuous. There are some individuals who doubtless do not realise that they have a hearing loss, especially if they live alone, but, in general, we simply do not want others to know that we are deaf and we put off seeking help. Deafness itself may be invisible but the impact of hearing loss is far more obvious. People with hearing loss can benefit from rehabilitative resources in order to compensate for hearing loss and overcome their associated problems.

Rejection of hearing problems and the need for hearing aids may be due to the stigma still attached to deafness. The general public tend to be ignorant of hearing loss and its effects. To them, hearing loss often appears as stupidity because of the communication difficulties that ensue. The hearing impaired person is therefore unwilling to accept, or tries to hide, their hearing loss. This in turn will often lead them to avoid situations which could be difficult and gradually their quality of life becomes more and more restricted.

1.1.4 Rejection

Sometimes it is the partner or another family member who first makes reference to a hearing problem, perhaps because the television is on very loud or because communicating with the hearing impaired person has become too much of a struggle. Pressure from others may lead the hearing impaired person to recognise that there is a problem – but this is not the same as fully accepting their hearing loss.

A problem occurs when a person wants to achieve something but does not know what series of actions to perform in order to achieve it. At first the hearing impaired individual often hopes that the problem will go away or be easily solvable, perhaps something such as a wax blockage with which the doctor or nurse can deal. The thought of having to wear a hearing aid is often unacceptable. The thought of having to wear two seems twice as bad as we have not educated the public to think of hearing aids in pairs like spectacles. Hearing aids are not considered attractive and, to overcome rejection, it is advantageous if the hearing aids can be as inconspicuous as possible *(see Figure 1.1)*. Types of hearing aids are introduced in Chapter 5. Small in-the-ear hearing aids and open fit mini behind-the-ear hearing aids are particularly helpful in improving acceptance amongst wearers.

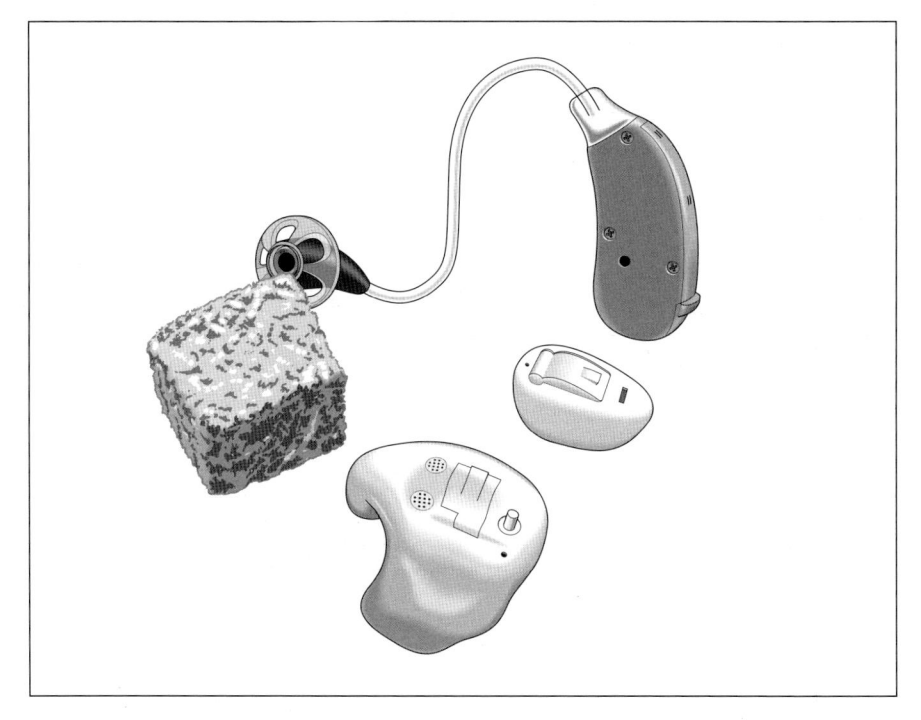

Figure 1.1 *Inconspicuous hearing aids (with a sugar cube for size comparison)*

1.2 EDUCATION

1.2.1 Attitude

The individual's attitude towards their hearing loss and to using hearing aids is an important factor in the amount of time that hearing aids are worn and to overall success in the rehabilitation process. Four main attitudinal types are often described, as shown in *Table 1.1*.

A negative attitude will generally result in a hearing loss that is, as far as possible, hidden and in hearing aids that are worn less than optimally. Miniaturisation and digitalisation of hearing aids have undoubtedly helped to reduce the stigma of wearing hearing aids and reducing costs and increased accessibility have further improved the situation. However, we still have a very long way to go before wearing a pair of hearing aids is accepted in the same way as wearing a pair of glasses.

Table 1.1 Attitude types

Type	Description
Type 1 'Mr Happy'	The client has a very positive attitude towards hearing aids and aural rehabilitation.
Type 2 'Mr Intrepid'	The client has an essentially positive attitude but with some complicating factors present, including an unfavourable past experience of using hearing aids.
Type 3 'Mr Grumpy'	The client has an essentially negative attitude but tries to co-operate.
Type 4 'Mr Impossible'	The client rejects hearing aids completely. This is the smallest group of clients, unfortunately rehabilitation is rarely successful here.

1.2.2 Acceptance

Regrettably, many people who come to have hearing aids fitted have not yet reached full acceptance of their loss. Often they blame other people for their inability to hear, for example thinking that other people are mumbling rather than accepting that their hearing could be at fault. Trialling a hearing aid may help the individual to realise what they are missing but if that person feels pushed into having hearing aids their motivation is likely to remain low. A positive attitude and self-motivation are important factors to rehabilitation success and counselling is often vital to their achievement. Counselling is covered in Chapter 8.

Expectations for hearing aids are not always realistic. 'Digital' hearing aids are often expected to be a 'magic cure' that will provide perfectly normal hearing. Many people are also under the impression that all hearing aids that are 'digital' are exactly the same. Education is needed from the very beginning. Explanation of the audiogram, of what digital means and of the advantages and limitations of hearing aids is generally a very worthwhile exercise both for the hearing impaired individual and for their spouse or partner. Amplification is covered in Chapter 5.

Hearing loss creates stress not only for the individual but also for their communication partners (family, friends and colleagues). The influence of the partner and family is often particularly important in getting the individual to seek help for their hearing problem but their importance does not end here. They can also be highly influential when hearing aids have been fitted. Once the individual has accepted that they have a hearing problem, they can, with the patience, understanding and support of their communication partner, develop a positive attitude to hearing aid use which will lead to a successful outcome. Where problems continue, counselling for the individual and the family may help in their resolution.

1.3 IMPAIRMENT, DISABILITY AND HANDICAP

The World Health Organisation (WHO) published an 'International Classification of Impairments, Disabilities and Handicaps' (World Health Organisation, 1994), which set out a model of the consequences of pathology and outlined differences between an impairment, a disability and a handicap:

- *An impairment* is any loss or abnormality of psychological, physiological or anatomical structure or function. Hearing impairment refers to a loss of hearing and is described in terms of decibels hearing loss.
- *A disability* is any restriction or lack of ability to perform an activity resulting from an impairment. Hearing disability is a functional limitation with regard to speech perception and is described in terms of a percentage disability.
- *A handicap* is the disadvantage that occurs because the disability limits the performance of roles considered normal for that person bearing in mind their age, gender and social situation. Handicap is difficult to quantify although attempts are made to do so by means of questionnaires.

Using this model, deafness can be viewed as a continuum in which pathological damage to the hearing system leads to impaired hearing. This results in a disability since speech is no longer fully understood. Finally, it is the degree to which the disability restricts the choices in a person's life that really causes the handicap. It should be noted that these definitions have been superseded because they are seen to relate to a medical model; this is discussed in Chapter 6. Notwithstanding this, these definitions may still be helpful in understanding the effects of hearing loss.

The World Health Organisation (2001) revised their classification in the 'International Classification of Functioning, Disability and Health'. This more recent classification abandons the word 'handicap' and expands the meaning of the word 'disability' to cover restrictions in activity. Although it is a more positive classification (Rehm et al, 1990) based on the effects of the disability not the cause, the original classification of impairment, disability and handicap continues to be widely used. Quantifying 'handicap' is particularly difficult because it will depend on the person's character, lifestyle, experiences and beliefs. Handicap is, to a great extent, subjective and therefore probably impossible to measure accurately. Certain tools exist, for example questionnaires, that do attempt to quantify it but all have their limitations. Also, since there is no single agreed or accepted measure for the determination of degree of handicap, making comparisons is difficult.

1.4 REHABILITATION

1.4.1 Definition

The Oxford Dictionary defines rehabilitation as:

Restoration to effectiveness or normal life by training etc., especially after imprisonment or illness. (Allen, 1991).

Rehabilitation is thus a process appropriate to those who have an acquired hearing loss and by which people can be reintegrated into society. It is not a term appropriate to those born deaf, who have never had speech and language skills to be 'restored'. The term 'habilitation', rather than rehabilitation, is more appropriate and generally used to mean teaching the skills for communication. Deafness from childhood is covered in Chapter 13.

1.4.2 The rehabilitation process

Rehabilitation is a process through which the disability caused by deafness is minimised. Communication skills are important to quality of life and rehabilitation seeks to reinstate successful communication between the hearing impaired person and their aural environment. Rehabilitation contributes to the likelihood of successful communication occurring by:

- Providing counselling to help overcome fears and other negative emotions, increasing acceptance of hearing loss and achieving realistic goals
- Increasing knowledge and understanding of hearing loss in the individual and their family and others
- Improving listening and other communication skills and supportive behaviours.

Rehabilitation is concerned with problem solving, see *Figure 1.2*. The process starts by identifying the problems through the case history, hearing assessment and discussion (covered in Chapter 4). It starts from the time the audiologist meets the new client. The process must be tailored to the individual to be of real value and must therefore start from an assessment of his or her needs. The audiologist must find what elements contribute to the client's communication problems and help them to accept their hearing impairment. No-one is likely to solve their problems until they have accepted their hearing loss and worked through any negative emotions. Once the situation has been analysed and the problem faced, help, advice and support must be planned and paced to meet the needs. Where the individual has unrealistic aspirations or a negative attitude, counselling may be required at an early stage to bring about changes that will allow the rehabilitation process to progress. Acquiring knowledge and understanding of hearing loss will help the client and their family to form realistic expectations of what is or is not possible.

Amplification is a part of the rehabilitation process and successful hearing aid use is usually an important pre-requisite to successful remediation. However, amplification is neither the beginning nor the end of the process.

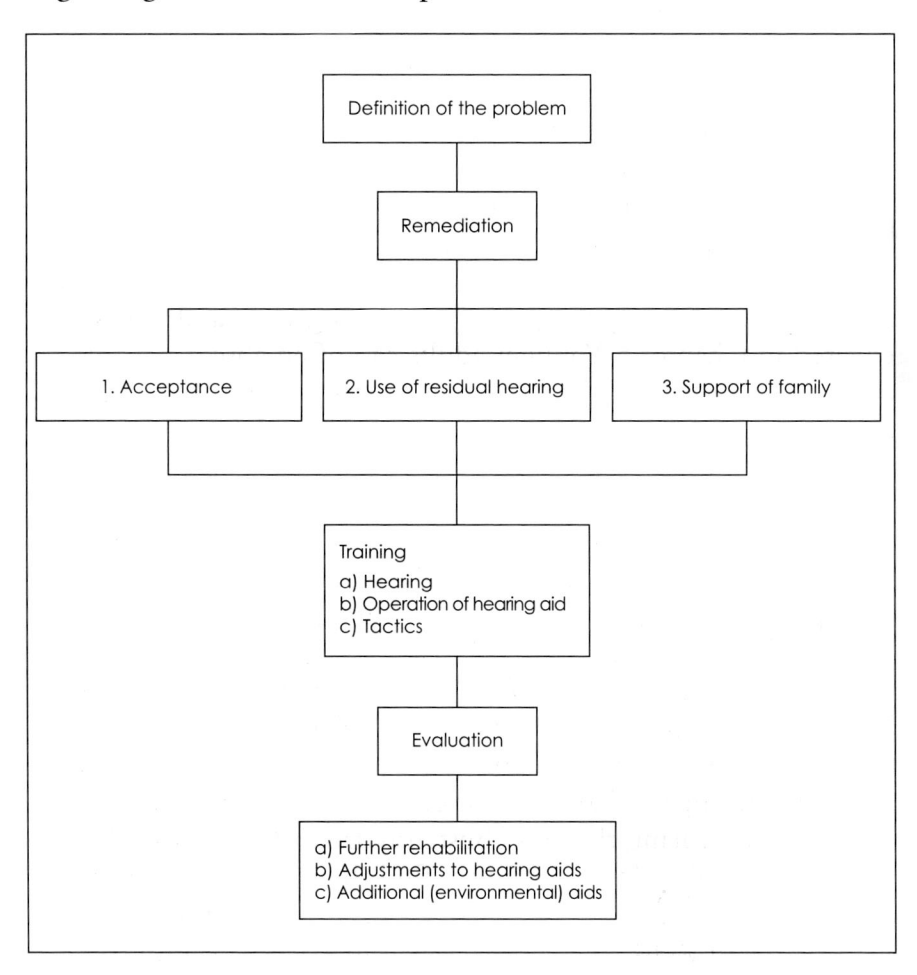

```
                    Definition of the problem
                              |
                         Remediation
                              |
        ┌─────────────────────┼─────────────────────┐
   1. Acceptance      2. Use of residual hearing    3. Support of family
        └─────────────────────┼─────────────────────┘
                              |
                         Training
                         a) Hearing
                         b) Operation of hearing aid
                         c) Tactics
                              |
                         Evaluation
                              |
                         a) Further rehabilitation
                         b) Adjustments to hearing aids
                         c) Additional (environmental) aids
```

Figure 1.2 *A simple problem-solving approach (Reproduced with kind permission of Maltby, 2002)*

Appropriate hearing aids have to be fitted and the client shown how to look after them and use them to best effect. Effective hearing aid use is affected by degree of hearing loss, attitude and family support but also by many other factors, the individual's health and age for example. If the individual has other disabilities these may also affect their ability to cope successfully with hearing aids. It could even be that hearing loss is the least of that person's worries, for example if they have a life-threatening condition. Or it may be that coping with two problems is just too much and one of the problems has to be 'solved' before the other can be faced, for example problems of vision (low vision aids, cataract operations, etc.) may need to be tackled prior to starting with hearing aids.

Information about the care of the hearing aid and aural hygiene will normally be given at the fitting stage and this is covered in Chapter 5. Younger adults can often absorb a great deal of information and also need much less rehabilitation than their older counterparts. Elderly adults tend to need to take things slowly as their attention span and ability to retain information is reduced. They may need longer and more repetition to absorb what is necessary. They may also need more practice to be able to handle the aid effectively and to be able to insert and remove it. The particular needs and problems of the elderly are covered in Chapter 3. Rehabilitation is usually undertaken over a number of sessions and it may be necessary to break the instructions into parts so that what is really important is given in the fitting session with less immediately important information imparted at a later session. Younger adults are often able to start wearing the aids constantly from the point of the first fitting whilst older adults may find their experience tiring and difficult. They may need to build up use more slowly and to use the aids in relatively easy listening environments until they have become used to wearing them. In any case, everyone should be warned against immediately 'trying the aids out' in the most difficult situations, such as in the pub or at meetings. Written material is advisable to support what has been taught, so that the individual can look things up later if they are uncertain or have forgotten.

Hearing aid usage may be built up gradually but the objective is normally to use the aids all (or at least most) of the day, whether the person is at home or away, in or out, at leisure or at work. There are many tactics that can be used to help improve the listening experience, which will be covered in Chapter 5. Tactics include even such simple things as speaking the hearing impaired person's name to attract their full attention before starting on the 'message', or repeating or rephrasing important points. The client can learn to be assertive and to take control in many listening situations. Ideally the hearing aids will eventually be viewed as a part of that person, to be put on every morning on arising and taken off only at bedtime. Of course this does not always happen but time of use certainly correlates with the benefit derived from hearing aids.

Auditory training and speech reading can increase communication ability by improving visual attention, speech discrimination, memory, integration of visual and auditory information and confidence and motivation. Auditory activities and repair strategies can be tailored to the individual's problems and can be practised in a safe environment. The degree of success following rehabilitation can be measured using a variety of tools to assess such parameters as satisfaction, benefit, reduction in handicap, hours of use and improvement in speech discrimination or threshold levels (aided). A description of some evaluation tools will be found in Chapter 10. Appropriate evaluation will often lead onto further rehabilitation.

Chapter 2
The Impact of Hearing Loss

2.1 POPULATION STUDIES

The total population in the United Kingdom is about sixty million. Almost nine million of these (approximately one in seven of the population) have impaired hearing. Just over 16% of the adult population of the United Kingdom have an average hearing loss of 25dBHL or more in the better ear, averaged over the frequency range 500Hz, 1kHz, 2kHz and 4kHz (Davis, 1995). Most of these could benefit from hearing aids, see *Figure 2.1*; yet only two million people have them and only 1.4 million people use them regularly. Hearing aids are not often requested where a hearing loss is less than 40dBHL. About 698,000 people are severely or profoundly deaf and about 450,000 of these cannot hear well enough to use a telephone, even if the volume is increased. About 7% of adults (3.3 million people) have visited their general practitioner about tinnitus. About 0.5% (230,000 people) have tinnitus so severely that it has a marked effect on their ability to lead a normal life.

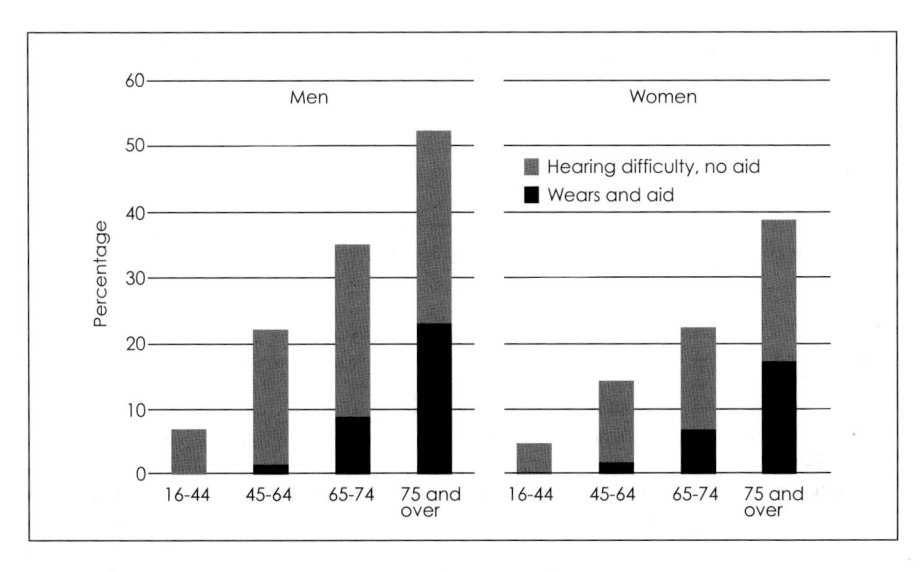

Figure 2.1 Hearing difficulty and the use of hearing aids: Great Britain 2002
(Source: National Statistics website www.statistics.gov.uk)

Nearly 6.5 million of those with impaired hearing are aged over sixty. The incidence of hearing loss increases with age. Approximately 42% of the over fifty year old age group are estimated to have a hearing loss; this increases to over 70% by the age of seventy (RNID, 2008) and virtually everyone by the age of eighty. Our population is ageing. We are having fewer children and we are living longer. Therefore the average age of the population is increasing and the number of deaf elderly is also increasing.

It is accepted generally that men lose their hearing in advance of women. The 2002/3 census indicates, as shown in *Figure 2.2*, that more men than women report hearing problems and the Health and Safety Executive use higher hearing levels as indicating normal or acceptable hearing for men than for women, see *Table 2.1*. Certainly over the age of forty, more men than women do become deaf. This is probably due to greater noise exposure rather than genetic factors. Similarly, after the age of eighty there are more women than men that are deaf due to the fact that there are more women than men by this age because they tend to have greater longevity.

Table 2.1 The Health and Safety Executive's normal or acceptable hearing levels by age
The scores in this table appear as a large number because they reflect the hearing levels at each of five frequencies added together

Age group	Sum of the hearing levels at 1kHz, 2kHz, 3kHz, 4kHz and 6kHz			
	Males		Females	
	Warning level	Referral level	Warning level	Referral level
18-24	51	95	46	78
25-29	67	113	55	91
30-34	82	132	63	105
35-39	100	154	71	119
40-44	121	183	80	134
45-49	142	211	93	153
50-54	165	240	111	176
55-59	190	269	131	204
60-64	217	296	157	235
65	235	311	175	255

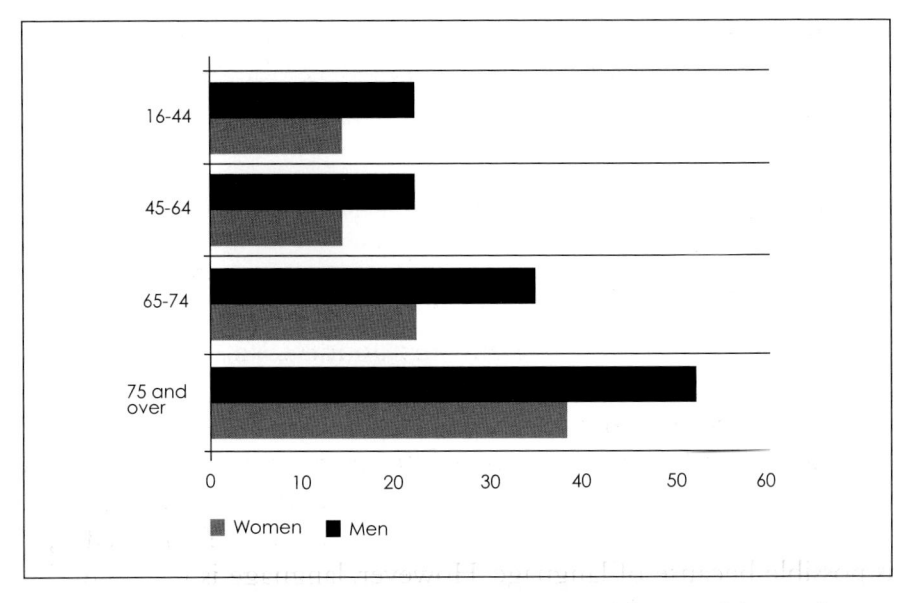

Figure 2.2 The percentage of men and women reporting some difficulty with hearing: by age (Source: National Statistics website www.statistics.gov.uk)

Approximately 50,000 deaf people in the United Kingdom use British Sign Language. Many people with severe or profound hearing loss also have other disabilities. Approximately 40% of those under sixty have additional needs but in the over sixty age group, as many as 77% have some additional disability. Many of these have dexterity or vision problems. There are approximately 23,000 deaf-blind people and about 16,000 of these are over seventy.

About one in every thousand children is born deaf (> 40dBHL) or goes deaf before they have acquired language. About one in every four thousand children is born profoundly deaf. Approximately 90% of deaf children are born to hearing parents. It is estimated that 840 children are born with moderate to profound hearing loss every year in the United Kingdom. In total there are over 30,000 deaf children, which is about 2% of the child and youth population and about 12,000 of these were born deaf. Approximately 23,000 children under sixteen wear hearing aids.

2.2 UNDERSTANDING SPEECH

2.2.1 The speech chain

Spoken language is an important part of normal human social behaviour. Wherever people live together, they develop a system of linguistic communication that is used to share ideas and experiences and to transmit knowledge from one generation to the next. Speaking, listening, reading and writing are all part of our social evolution. Education, the passing on of knowledge, is possible because of language. However, language is not a good medium for giving instructions and is not thought to have developed for this purpose (Aitchison, 2000). Reading and writing are language-based and closely related to talking and listening, so that once we perceive and identify written words we are usually able to understand their meaning.

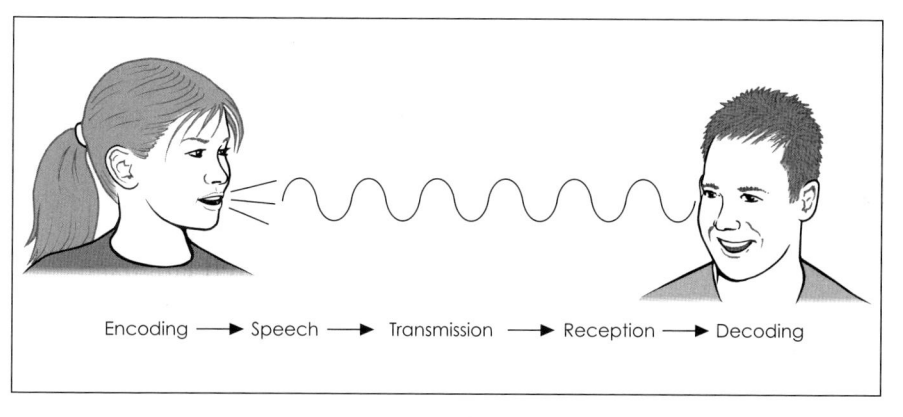

Figure 2.3 The speech chain

Communication through language is a two-way process, between a speaker who transmits the message and a listener who receives the message. It involves a number of elements, commonly referred to as the 'speech chain', see *Figure 2.3*. For the communication process to be successful the chain must be complete. The speaker must have a message to convey, based on the present or on memory or imagination. The speaker must then encode the thoughts in language and use motor skills to program and transmit them. The spoken message must be received by the listener who must perceive, recognise and decode it, in order to understand it.

When the speech message reaches the listener's ear, it travels through the outer and middle ears, see *Figure 2.4*, to reach the inner ear where the sound is coded into its individual frequency components. The auditory nerve carries this information to the auditory cortex in the brain, where conscious perception of the sound occurs and we hear. Complex processing of the auditory signal occurs at points along the auditory nerve and within the auditory cortex. Using previously learned experience, the brain subconsciously detects important messages and extracts them from unimportant background noise. Recognition of speech relies on memories of sequences of sounds, which is undertaken in Wernicke's area. However, for comprehension to occur, words not only have to be recognised but their meaning also has to be understood.

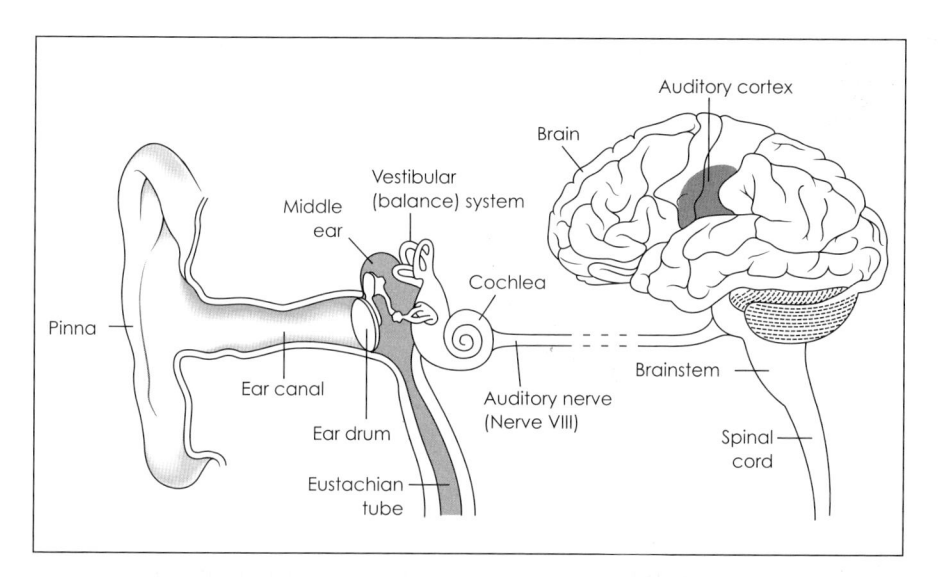

Figure 2.4 *The journey through the ear*

2.2.2 The varying effect of a hearing loss

The effect of a hearing loss on the individual depends on a number of factors, such as:

i) The type of hearing loss
ii) The degree of hearing loss
iii) The age the loss occurred
iv) The speed of onset
v) Whether the loss affects one ear (unilateral) or both (bilateral).

i) The type of hearing loss

Hearing loss is common and may be conductive or sensorineural or both (mixed loss). Conductive hearing loss can often be medically or surgically treated; sensorineural loss is rarely treatable apart from with the use of hearing aids. If medical or surgical treatment is not possible hearing aids, within a rehabilitative programme, can help to overcome the problems.

Conductive hearing loss is caused by some problem in the outer or middle ears which prevents, to some degree, the sound travelling through the normal route. There are many causes of conductive hearing loss such as otitis media, otosclerosis or even simply a wax blockage. Otitis media ('glue ear') is a particularly common cause of conductive hearing loss in children, which can slow language development and/or education. Much conductive loss is temporary and will resolve itself or can be treated medically or surgically.

Conductive loss typically presents with an audiogram that is either 'flat' across the frequency range or that is worse in the low frequencies, see *Figure 2.5*. A conductive loss tends to affect volume rather than clarity and the person with a conductive loss often speaks quietly because they tend to hear their own voice louder than that of other people. The reason for this is that a person hears their own voice partly by air conduction (the normal route for sound via the ear canal) and partly by bone conduction (direct to the cochlea via the bones of the skull). With a conductive loss, the air conduction route is blocked but the bone conduction route is working normally. The person's own voice is therefore heard clearly by bone conduction, whilst other people's voices and background noise are reduced in volume.

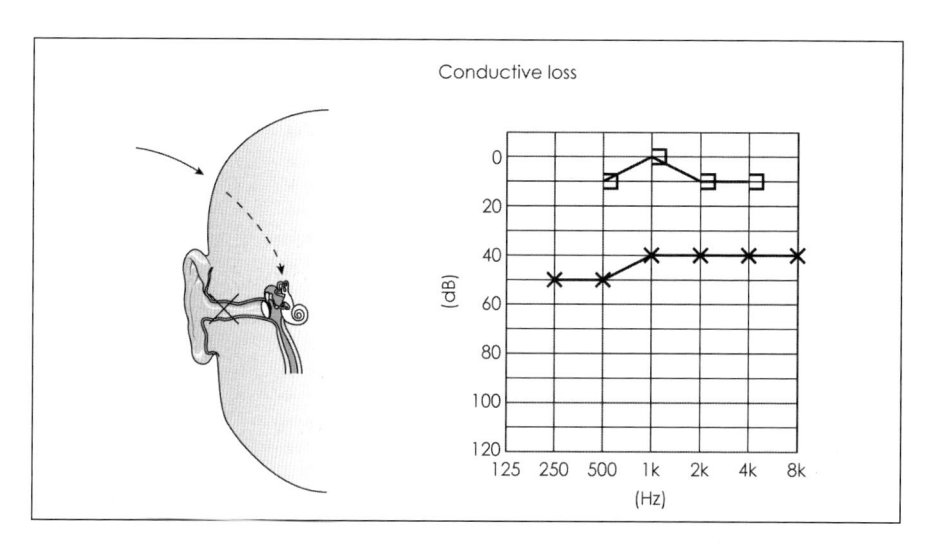

Figure 2.5 Conductive hearing loss

Sensorineural hearing loss is a problem in or beyond the cochlea, caused by, for example, excessive noise, ototoxic drugs, viral infections or high blood pressure. The most common 'cause' of sensorineural hearing loss is presbyacusis, which is the hearing loss of old age. This is not really a single cause but rather is hearing loss due to various problems associated with ageing. In fact, the most common single cause is excessive noise. In some cases hearing loss is present from birth, due to causes such as German measles (rubella) in the pregnancy or heredity.

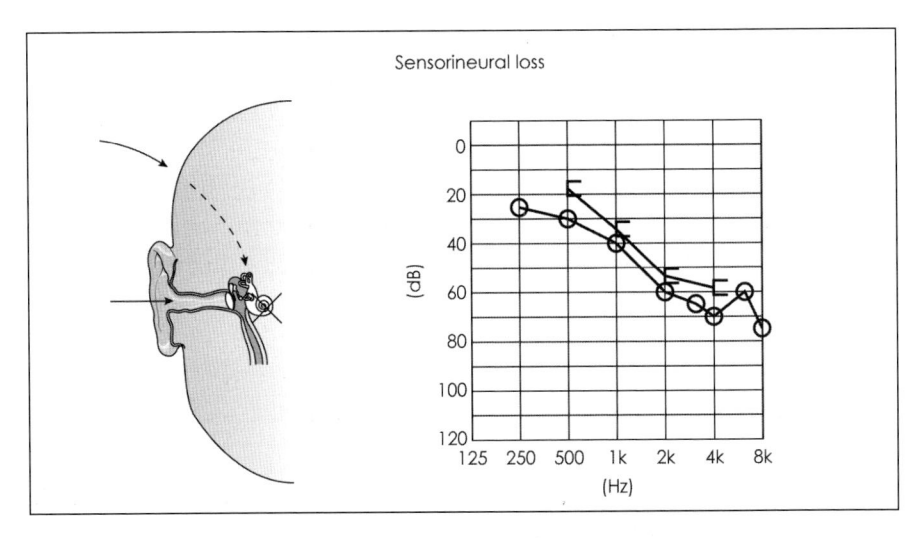

Figure 2.6 Sensorineural hearing loss

Sensorineural hearing loss is usually a permanent problem and the hearing loss is commonly worse in the higher frequencies, see *Figure 2.6*. It is these high frequencies that particularly affect the perception of consonants. Unfortunately, consonants provide the most important distinguishing factors between similar words and the loss of consonants is detrimental to understanding speech.

People with sensorineural hearing loss tend to speak loudly because they cannot hear themselves clearly. In addition to reduced hearing sensitivity, they may also have more subtle changes to their hearing ability, such as difficulties with the separation of sounds that are close in time or pitch, and therefore simple amplification of sound may not produce increased clarity.

Another very common problem with sensorineural loss is recruitment. This is an abnormal perception of loudness in which weak sounds are too quiet, whilst stronger sounds very rapidly become too loud and it is caused by outer hair cell damage within the cochlea, see *Figure 2.7*. The function of the outer hair cells is to amplify the level of quiet sounds by a mechanical process and where there are reduced or missing areas of outer hair cells they are not able to function properly, resulting in weak sounds that are inaudible. Since stronger sounds do not require extra amplification, the loss of outer hair cells will not affect the louder sounds in this way and so they may still be heard as loud, despite the hearing loss. Indeed, many of us are aware of deaf people who fail to hear when we speak normally but then, when we raise our voices, accuse us of shouting! This is due to recruitment through loss of hair cell function.

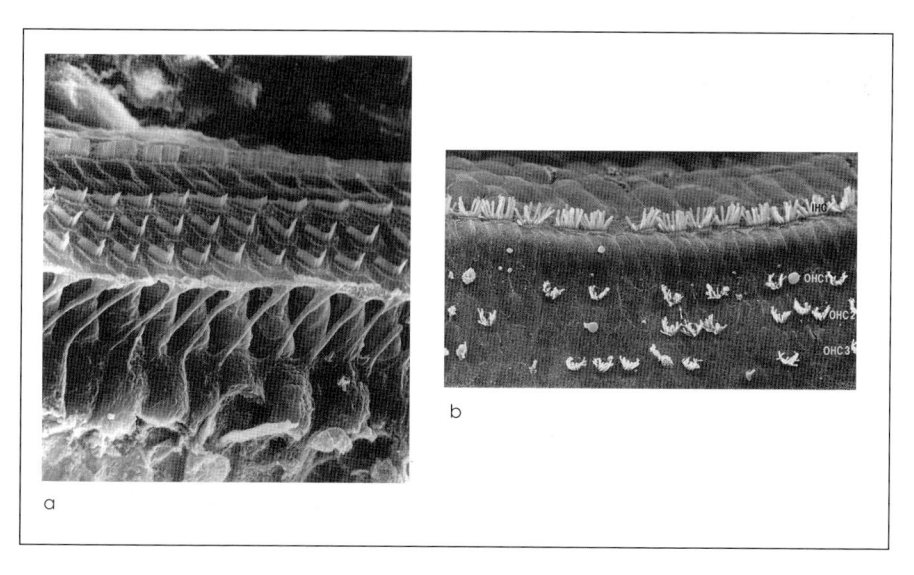

Figure 2.7 *Hair cell damage (a) Normal (b) Damaged (Reproduced with kind permission of Widex Engström)*

Most sensorineural hearing loss is due to hair cell damage in the cochlea. Uncommonly, hearing loss may also be due to retrocochlear causes, that is damage to the auditory nerve or hearing centres of the brain. This, for example, could be due to a tumour or as the result of an accident affecting the head. Retrocochlear losses may cause very poor speech perception and comprehension and are usually not helped by hearing aids.

ii) The degree of hearing loss

The extent of a hearing loss is usually described as an average in decibels, often taken over the five frequencies 250Hz, 500Hz, 1kHz, 2kHz and 4kHz. Audiometric descriptors based on this five frequency average of the pure tone hearing threshold levels may be used to describe the average hearing level as follows:

- 20-40dBHL: Mild hearing loss
- 41-70dBHL: Moderate hearing loss
- 71-95dBHL: Severe hearing loss
- Over 95dBHL: Profound hearing loss.

Average hearing threshold levels of less than 20dB do not necessarily imply normal hearing, neither do averages imply any particular configuration of hearing loss. Additional terms may be used to add clarity, as for example 'a mild high-frequency hearing loss'.

The degree of hearing loss is obviously an important factor in the amount of difficulty encountered. A mild degree of hearing loss will generally cause minimal difficulty whilst a severe or profound loss is likely to result in major communication problems.

iii) The age at which the hearing loss occurred

A child who is born deaf will have difficulty in learning spoken language, the degree of difficulty relating mainly to the degree of the hearing impairment. This also applies to any child who goes deaf before acquiring language (pre-lingual), which is generally taken to be before the age of about two. Most people go deaf later in life when their speech and language skills are developed (post-lingual).

Social problems and reduced quality of life can affect hearing impaired people of all ages. However the degree of impact will be related to social, educational and employment circumstances. Communication difficulties will impact upon learning and, if education is not complete, learning will be slower and more effortful. Employment opportunities may be restricted and communication problems may affect work tasks and relationships. Elderly adults usually find greater difficulty in conversing with younger people than their own age group who understand and often share their problems. Elderly people may also have difficulty in handling hearing aids and in learning new strategies.

iv) The speed of onset

Gradual hearing loss, as is common in old age, occurs slowly and allows the person to make adjustments, often without even realising it. For some considerable time (several years) the loss may not be accepted or may even go unnoticed. As high-frequency sounds are generally lost first, speech gradually becomes less intelligible. It is very common to hear an older person say that they 'can hear but not understand' which is a typical result of high-frequency hearing loss. Listening becomes a struggle and communication starts to break down. Participating in conversations becomes uncertain, unpredictable and stressful. Misunderstandings are commonplace and the individual may feel bewildered and confused and be unable to respond appropriately. Communication difficulties with family and colleagues are common with feelings of frustration on both sides. Family and colleagues may view the hearing impaired person as awkward because he hears some things and therefore may seem to 'hear when he wants to'. In general, hearing loss is frustrating for others. Having to repeat things a number of times is irritating and often ends in the response 'Oh, it doesn't matter' with the deaf person being, or at least feeling, left out.

When a person loses their hearing traumatically they do not have the opportunity to adapt gradually. They are likely to experience shock, bewilderment, denial, anger, grief and depression before they can finally accept the situation. Unless the loss is minor, they are likely to suffer immediate disruption of their ability to communicate and long-lasting changes to their home and social life and to their employment and educational prospects, with accompanying loss of confidence, social withdrawal and depression.

v) Unilateral or bilateral hearing loss

When hearing loss is discussed, it is generally referred to as deafness in both ears (bilaterally). A bilateral hearing loss can result in all the problems mentioned in relation to deafness. A unilateral loss, where only one ear is affected, will give rise to less severe problems. The unilaterally impaired person can manage fairly well in most situations by making minor adjustments such as turning towards the sound source. In general, the public at large tend to think that unilateral hearing is adequate. This is not true as the two ears work together to utilise small differences in the time, frequency and phase between sounds reaching each ear. These small differences facilitate localisation of sounds and separation of speech or other meaningful signals from background or unwanted noise. A unilaterally hearing impaired person will therefore have:

- Difficulty in hearing in background noise
- Difficulty hearing in groups
- Difficulty in localising sounds.

2.2.3 Tinnitus

Tinnitus is noises in the head or ears (without an external source) and is common with hearing loss. If tinnitus is troublesome it should be treated. Medical or surgical treatment is not often possible but masking is often effective, particularly when combined with psychological help. Masking is the introduction of another less intrusive sound which can reduce the severity of the tinnitus. One approach used is Tinnitus Retraining Therapy (TRT) which helps the individual to cope with the problem by counselling to allay fears in conjunction with a low-level noise generating device (a masker). The noise produced by the masker is not intended to completely mask (cover) the tinnitus but helps to decrease the brain's sensitivity to the tinnitus. Relaxation training and counselling can help to improve the effectiveness of the tinnitus retraining programme.

2.2.4 Public attitudes to deafness

The public at large has a stereotyped view of deafness. Traditionally deafness is a suitable subject for jokes and there is a general misconception that if you are deaf you do not hear anything or you hear all sounds equally poorly. There is therefore a lack of understanding and empathy and even a feeling that deaf people can hear when they want to and could do better if they tried harder. People with all degrees of deafness may encounter discrimination when looking for work, while at their jobs, or when socialising with normally hearing people.

Born deaf people are often viewed by the hearing population as being 'deaf and dumb'. The word 'dumb' is commonly used to mean stupid and there is a tendency to equate deafness with stupidity. Many of the symptoms of deafness, such as not answering when spoken to, answering inappropriately, using incorrect pitch and having impaired speech, are unfortunately ones that are also associated with impaired cognitive ability. This tends to add to the misconception.

Deafness is also widely associated with ageing. In our present society, both old age and mental disorder carry stigma. A sense of embarrassment and shame prevents people from explaining that they are deaf or seeking help. Deafness is regarded as a disability to be hidden. In general, we view deafness as a disability that causes an undesirable disruption of life. Our goal is therefore to change things so that life can return to normal, although this is rarely a realistic goal.

2.2.5 The Deaf community

People with acquired deafness generally want to remain part of the hearing community and be able to maintain their hearing relationships, their oral social interactions and their position in the hearing world. Many of those who are born deaf prefer to separate themselves from the hearing world as far as possible and they become part of the Deaf community with its own language and culture.

The Deaf (written with a capital D) community is a minority cultural group of people who use a sign language as their first language and who hold social and cultural norms which are distinctly different from those of the surrounding hearing community. The Deaf do not see themselves as disabled but as members of a cultural or language minority. Sign language is a form of manual communication with its own structure which is different from spoken language. British sign language (BSL) is the most widely used sign language in the UK. The Deaf community includes any person who identifies themselves as a member of the Deaf community, for example hearing relatives and spouses and signing friends and colleagues could be included as part of the Deaf community.

Although signed communication is the primary language of the Deaf community, most Deaf people have some knowledge of their country's dominant language. Knowledge of both the dominant language and sign language is known as *bilingualism*.

Most people with hearing loss can benefit from hearing aids. Although some Deaf people choose not to use hearing aids, there are very few people who have such a profound loss that hearing aids are of no real benefit. Someone with profound deafness may be a candidate for cochlear implants, however not all Deaf people would wish to embrace this technology. Cochlear implants are a highly specialised type of hearing aid in which the damaged structures of the cochlea are bypassed by electrodes placed within the cochlea. Normally an intact auditory nerve is required but other implants do also exist that can be placed beyond the auditory nerve, on the cochlear nucleus, see *Figure 2.8*, or on the brainstem, see *Figure 2.9*.

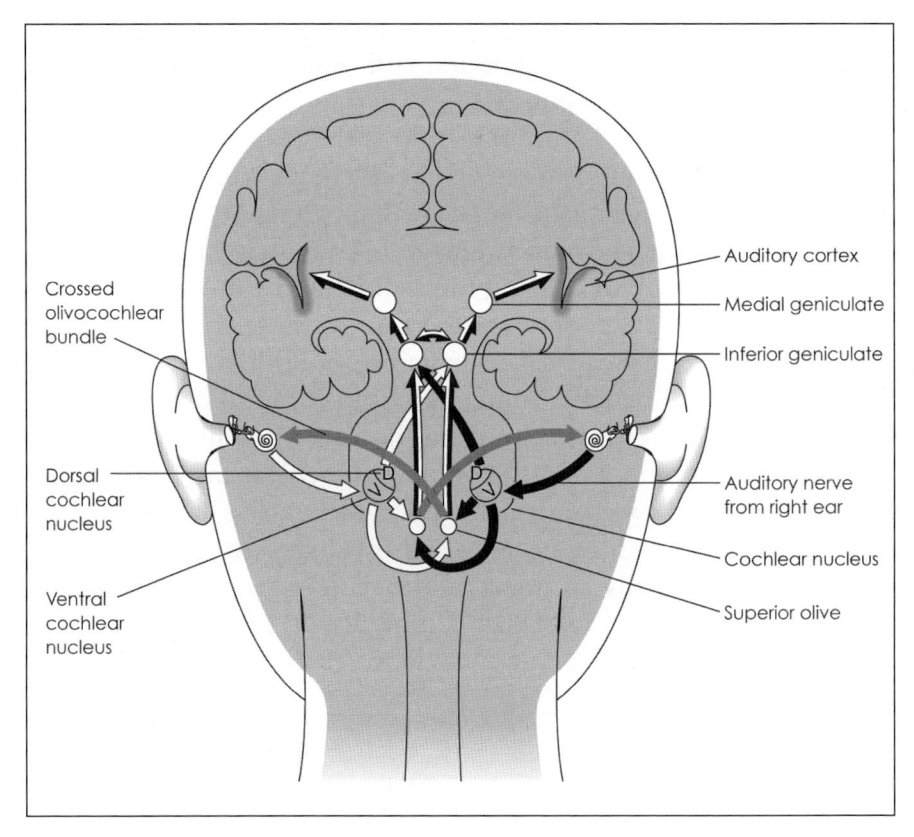

Figure 2.8 *The major auditory pathways of the brain*

2.2.6 Disruption of the speech message

The speech medium is, in general, a hardy one and tolerant of noise, distortion, accent and other interference. However, a break at any point in the chain will disrupt the message. Such a break could be due to one of many things, for example a foreign language, an inappropriate language level, a sensory impairment (e.g. vision or hearing), lack of concentration, differences in culture or experience, poor listening environment, learning difficulty, or even a specific language disorder, see *Table 2.2*.

The Impact of Hearing Loss

Much of the study of the neuroanatomical basis of spoken language (that is the study of Neurolinguistics) has been based on observation of the effects of brain damage in specific areas, see *Table 2.3*.

Table 2.2 Specific speech and language disorders

Name of Disorder	Difficulty
Agnosia (auditory)	Inability to recognise sounds, despite normal hearing and no significant loss of memory.
Anomia	Difficulty finding words and the person will tend to omit words or use inappropriate ones to fill the gap. Anomia is a primary symptom in all aphasia.
Aphasia	Inability to produce and/or comprehend language due to brain damage or abnormal development.
Apraxia/ Dyspraxia (of speech)	Neurological inability or difficulty in using the muscles of articulation to coordinate sequences of speech movements.
Agrammartism	Difficulty in using and understanding grammar, for example grammatical markers such as –ed or –ing.
Autism	Impaired social interaction and communication with restricted and repetitive behaviours.
Developmental language disorder	Abnormality in the development of language use and/or understanding with no obvious cause.

Table 2.2 Specific speech and language disorders continued

Dysarthria	Physical difficulty in using the muscles of articulation (mouth, tongue, throat and larynx).
Dysfluency	Stumbling over speech making it difficult to understand (includes stuttering and stammering).
Dysphonia	Disorder of voice.

In about 95% of right-handed people and about 70% of left-handed people, both speech production and perception are lateralised in the left side of the brain. The left side of the brain is specialised for sequential stimuli including the control of sequences of sounds and words, whilst the right side is more specialised for the analysis of space and geometrical form where elements tend to be present at the same time. The right hemisphere is concerned with rhythm and stress (prosody), selecting and organising what we are going to say, expression and recognition of emotion in the voice, and memory.

Table 2.3 Areas of the brain and their function

Part of brain	Includes	Controls
Hind-brain	Medulla oblongata	Respiration; blood pressure; heart beat
	Reticular formation	Alertness
	Pons and cerebellum	Muscular and positional information
Mid-brain	Thalamus	Attention; memory; emotions Links to cerebral cortex for higher processing
	Hypothalamus	Appetite; thirst; sexual arousal
	Limbic system	Evaluates sensory information and controls resulting behaviour; memory
Cerebrum	Basal ganglia	Motor co-ordination
	Cortex:	See below:
	i) Frontal lobes	Speech co-ordination; motor co-ordination; behaviour planning
	ii) Temporal lobes	Integration of senses; visuo-spatial processing, smell and hearing; language
	iii) Occipital and iv) Parietal lobes	Integration of sensory information; interpretation of visual stimuli

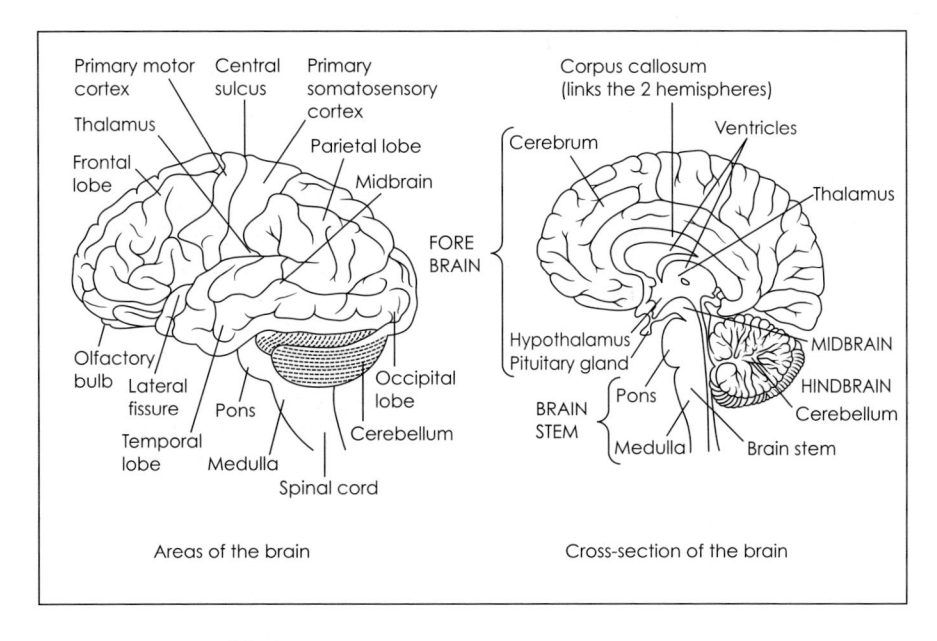

Figure 2.9 *Areas of the brain*

Brain damage in specific areas of the brain (see *Figure 2.9*) can result in speech and language problems. Damage to the frontal lobes is likely to cause aphasia, for example Broca's aphasia is due to damage in Broca's area, which is involved with speech production. Speech involves rapid movements of the tongue, lips and jaw which must be co-ordinated and Broca's area is thought to contain memories of the sequences of movements needed to articulate words. Someone with Broca's aphasia will have poor articulation, lack fluency and have comprehension that is much better than their expression. They will have difficulty in finding the words they need, especially grammatical or function words and difficulty with carrying out sequences of instructions. Nevertheless their speech will be meaningful. Damage to Wernicke's area, which is in the temporal lobes and concerned with speech perception, results in poor comprehension and fluent but meaningless speech. This problem is called receptive aphasia. Individuals with damage to this area tend to have difficulty in recognising spoken words, understanding the meaning of words and converting thoughts into words.

Deaf individuals who are fluent in sign language use a grammar that is spatial in nature and much of the grammar is indicated by movements that modify the signs. Nevertheless, aphasia in deaf people is caused by damage to the left hemisphere not by damage in the area responsible for spatial perception!

Chapter 3
The Ageing Process

3.1 'TYPICAL' OLD AGE

Ageing people should know that their lives are not mounting and unfolding but that an inexorable inner process forces the contraction of life. For a young person it is almost a sin – and certainly a danger – to be too much occupied with himself; but for the ageing person it is a duty and a necessity to give serious attention to himself.
(Jung, 1933)

Ageing is a continuous process from birth to death. In our society we value youth but not old age, see *Figure 3.1*. Typically we ignore positive aspects of old age and view it only as a period of deterioration and decline.

Ageing causes a number of physiological changes that affect both looks and functioning. The skin wrinkles and appears thinner and more translucent and becomes less sensitive, brown patches or 'age spots' appear, nails thicken and hair turns grey. Muscles lose their mass and tone, which is noticeable as loose skin under the arms, sagging breasts and thinner legs and arms. Elderly people also lose height as the cartilage between the vertebrae loses its resilience. A general decline in cellular activity occurs that leads to a slowing down of all the organ systems. An elderly person may therefore have to deal not only with changing looks but also with a number of disabilities, such as failing hearing and eyesight, loss of motor skills and cognitive changes.

'Old age' also involves an increasingly wide age range with significant differences across it. It is sometimes helpful to divide the period we call 'old age' into a number of shorter periods because there is a wide difference between the abilities of someone of fifty and a person of eighty, for example. One possible division might be:

- Young-old (aged 45-64)
- Old (aged 65-74)
- Old-old (aged 75 or more).

However, chronological age can be misleading as some people do decline rapidly, but for most the changes are gradual. Chronological age also fails to reflect how a person feels and that they may feel a different age at different times of the day or with different activities or varying levels of stress. Although we categorise people by their chronological age it may tell us little about the person's abilities or feelings. There are wide individual differences. It may therefore be useful to consider:

- Biological age (how old is the person in years?)
- Psychological age (how well adapted is the person?)
- Social age (how does the person compare with their social group?).

Individual differences can be influenced by both genetic and environmental factors. Indeed, some of the changes that we consider to be a normal part of ageing are due, at least in part, to lifestyle or disease. Genetic factors undoubtedly have a great influence but environmental factors, such as exercise, diet, smoking and stress, can also impact upon the ageing process and, of course, on life span itself.

The ageing process 39

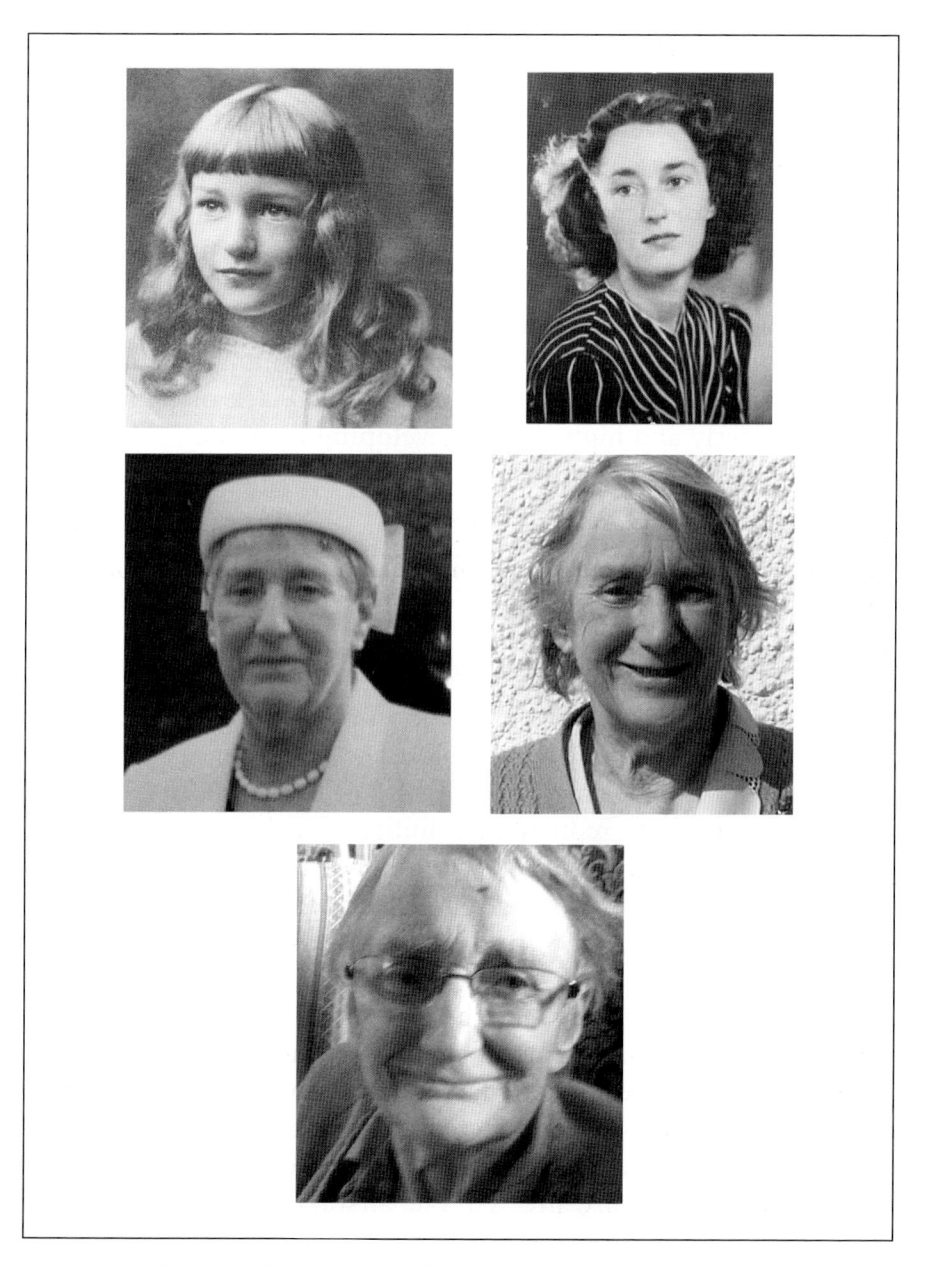

Figure 3.1 The process of ageing: Frances from 9 to 90

3.2 THE PHYSICAL EFFECTS OF AGEING

3.2.1 The endocrine and the immune systems

Hormonal changes play a part in ageing. Loss of oestrogen in women at the menopause creates increased risk of cardiovascular disease, reduced bone mass and cognitive impairments. Reduced testosterone in men may cause reduced muscle strength, anaemia and mood disturbances. Other hormones also diminish in old age, for example, insulin production declines by as much as half by age 80 and this, combined with poor diet and lack of exercise, puts the elderly at a high risk of developing diabetes.

The body's response to infections is reduced by age-related changes to the immune system and, as well as increased vulnerability to illness generally, this can also result in the re-emergence of latent infections, such as tuberculosis.

3.2.2 The musculo-skeletal system

As we age, the transport and absorption of calcium and vitamin D decreases. Calcium is gradually lost and bone density declines, which results in an increased likelihood of broken bones. The vertebrae can calcify, reducing flexibility so making bending difficult and causing postural changes. The cartilage of the joints may become diseased or wear away; arthritis (degenerative inflammation of the joints) may develop. Risk of fractures increases.

Muscles start to atrophy, which results in a general loss of strength and slower movement and an increased risk of falling. Specific problems occur in:

- *The lungs.* The ability to breathe deeply, cough and expel carbon dioxide are affected. The airways and lung tissue become less elastic and cilia activity declines. As a result

oxygen exchange decreases. Lack of oxygen can not only reduce stamina but also increase anxiety.
- *The gastro-intestinal and urinary systems.* Production of hydrochloric acid, digestive enzymes and saliva decreases, which can result in impaired swallowing and impaired digestion and absorption of foods. Reduced muscle tone can lead to constipation and to bladder incontinence. Urination is more frequent and more urgent. The filtering function of the kidneys slows, which results in medication remaining for longer in the bloodstream and possible over-medication.
- *The heart.* Most heart cells (myocytes) cannot regenerate. With age the heart muscle begins to atrophy making it weaken, stiffen and lose pumping capacity. The walls of the blood vessels lose their elasticity and the vessels may become blocked, so the blood flow to the body is reduced. As a result, if the elderly person gets up too quickly they may feel dizzy and stumble or appear confused for a few seconds, although in general reduced blood flow does not greatly affect daily life. As with many of the features of ageing, however, one thing tends to lead to another and reduced blood flow results in reduced oxygen which leads to reduced kidney and liver function and less cellular nourishment. The elderly person, especially beyond the age of about eighty, has reduced stamina, a slower rate of healing and reduced response to environmental stress (such as toxins, ultraviolet light, heat, cold, etc.) and is more at risk of strokes and heart failure.

Changes tend to be gradual and most elderly people adapt to the changes and continue to function well in their everyday life; the changes generally only cause significant problems when the elderly person is in an unfamiliar environment or under stress.

3.2.3 Sensory changes

i) Hearing

The reduced hearing sensitivity of old age is known as *presbyacusis*. Hearing deteriorates most in the high frequencies. Within the speech range, the high frequencies are responsible for speech understanding, whereas the lower frequencies provide the volume of speech. Changes that occur in the inner ear are largely responsible for the reduction in high frequency hearing although the whole of the auditory system undergoes age-related changes. The high frequency hearing range may reduce by as much as 80Hz every six months from about the age of about 40 to 45 but the loss is not really noticed until the range used for hearing speech is affected. As old age advances, the rate at which hearing is lost increases so that by the age of 80 - 85 years, a deterioration rate of almost 2dB per year at 6kHz may be expected, whilst at 1kHz the rate of loss is much less, about 0.35dB annually (Keay and Murray, 2007).

In the outer ear, loss of elasticity in the skin and cartilage may result in enlarged soft flaccid pinnae and collapsed ear canals (sometimes a particular problem when testing hearing as the earphones can cause a collapse that was not apparent before). Reduced elasticity can cause difficulties with the fit of an earmould or an in-the-ear hearing aid. Thinning and drying skin makes tissue damage more likely and healing is slower in the elderly. Extra care is needed for these reasons and if a poor fit is ignored it can result in the inability to wear a hearing aid for a considerable period.

In the middle ear, changes may include reduced elasticity, atrophied muscles and arthritic joints, although these do not necessarily result in a conductive hearing loss. Hearing loss is most affected by the changes in the inner ear, see *Figure 3.2*, where there may be degenerative changes to:

- *The hair cells and supporting cells.* Reduced sensory messages are sent to the brain (particularly affecting high frequency hearing).
- *The nerve pathways and brain* (especially the brain stem and auditory cortex). These changes may be physical and neurochemical. They cause *central auditory processing disorders* in which the ability to understand speech is considerably worse than the audiometric levels (response to pure tones) would suggest. The cochlea may be relatively intact in this type of loss, in which case amplification is not always helpful. Some central auditory involvement (i.e. within the brain or central nervous system) is increasingly common beyond the age of eighty.
- *The stria vascularis.* These changes may be the cause of genetic hearing loss usually occurring around the age of thirty to forty. Metabolic changes occur as nutrition to the cochlea is reduced. The resultant hearing loss is typically around 50dB and flat across the frequency range.
- *The tectorial and basilar membranes.* The membranes may stiffen causing mechanical changes within the cochlea.

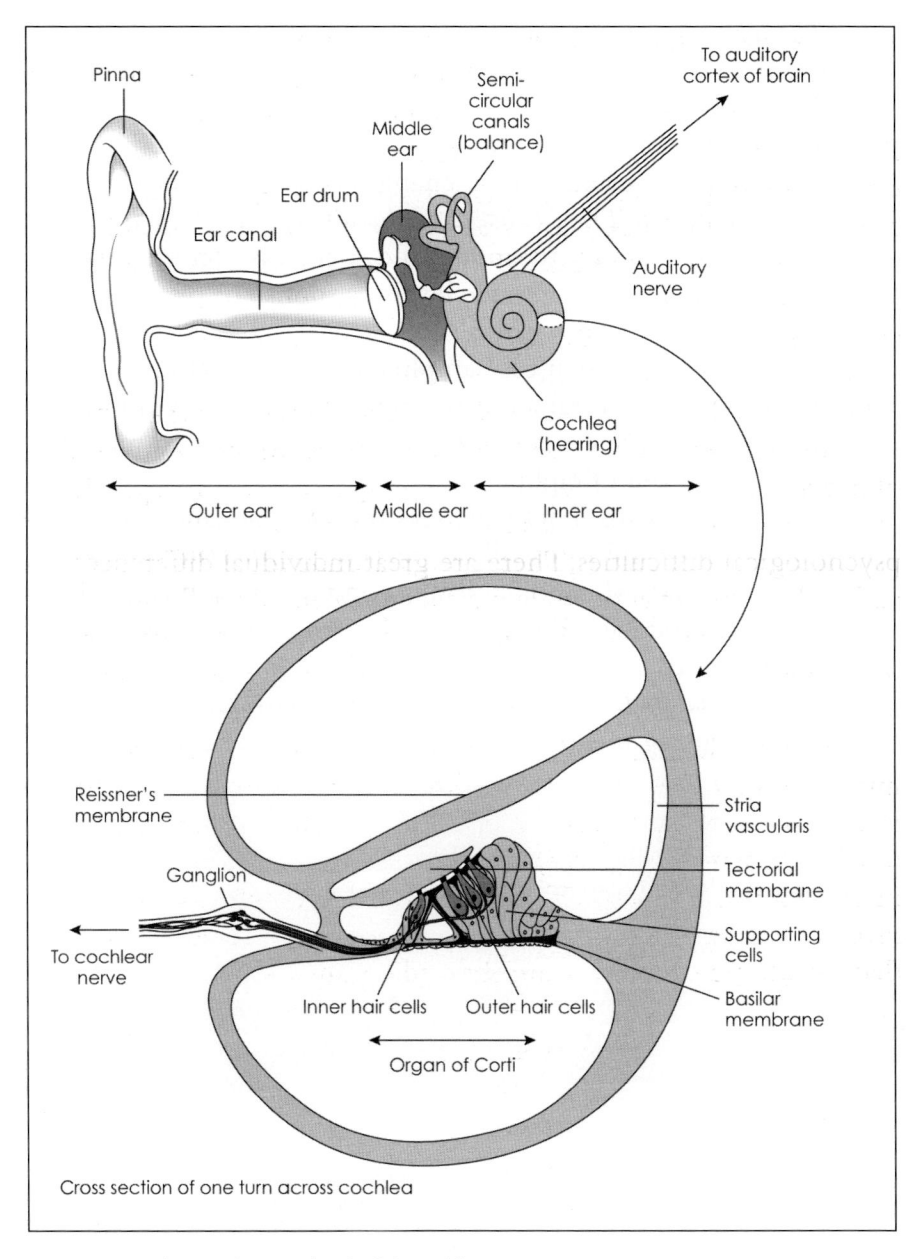

Figure 3.2 *The ear showing detail of the cochlea*

The hearing loss in presbyacusis is typically sensorineural and mainly high frequency, see *Figure 3.3*. The loss tends to be gradual but the rate of its progress increases with increasing age. Presbyacusis is not due simply to ageing, rather it involves the effects of living a long life. There are predisposing factors, such as high blood pressure, high cholesterol and arteriosclerosis but basically the longer the life, the more the person is likely to have been exposed to environmental factors such as ototoxic medications, noise, etc. The effects of ageing itself are difficult (if not impossible) to differentiate from the effects of environmental factors. The resulting condition, *presbyacusis*, may lead to impaired auditory sensitivity, temporal processing (speed of processing), temporal discrimination (gap detection), speech discrimination, auditory recall and associated social and psychological difficulties. There are great individual differences and audiograms may be widely different. Men generally appear to have worse hearing loss (above 1kHz) than women but this too could be due to a variety of factors, not necessarily genetic, for example exposure to noisier work or hobbies.

Hearing loss is usually accompanied by poorer speech understanding. It is the reduced ability to communicate which is most debilitating and frustrating. It is socially disabling and usually compounded by failing vision so that supportive visual information is also lost. Where there is central auditory involvement, speech understanding may be considerably worse than would be expected from the audiogram.

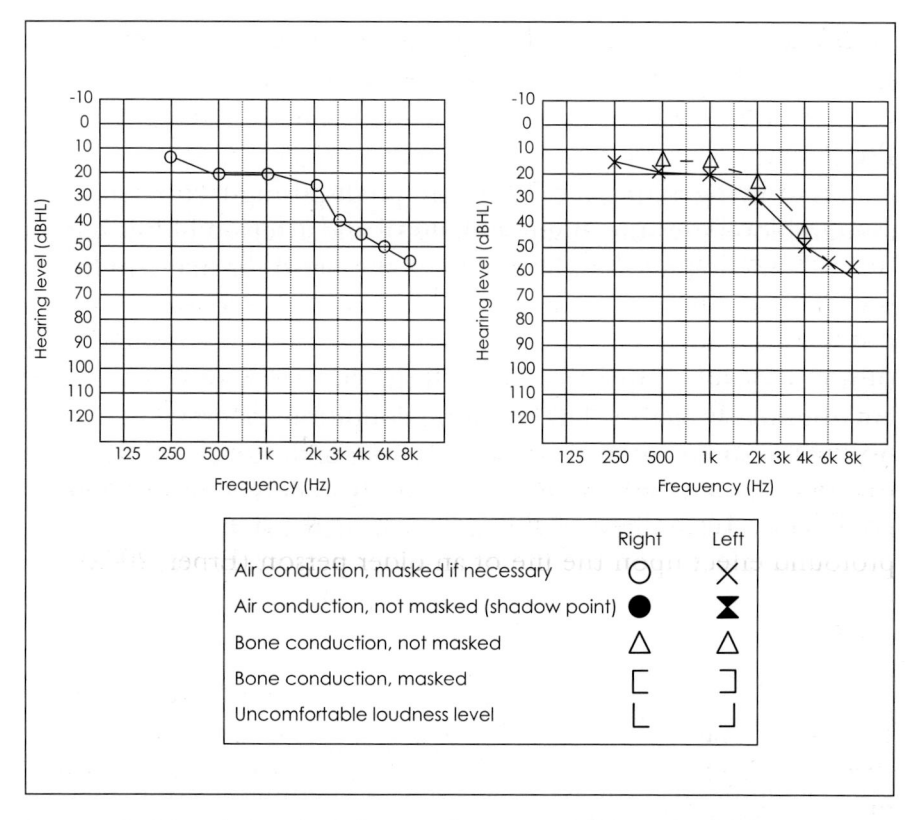

Figure 3.3 *Average hearing levels due to presbyacusis in 65 old year females (Demeester et al, 2009)*

ii) Vision

From about the age of forty, pupil size decreases – the eye cannot therefore adjust as well to changing amounts of light; more time is needed to adjust and more light is needed to see clearly. An elderly person may need three or four times more illumination than younger adults.

With increasing age, the lens of the eye thickens and yellows, resulting in increased sensitivity to glare, decreased depth perception (making it difficult to judge the height of steps and curbs) and more difficulty distinguishing between blues and greens and between pinks and yellows. Similar shades of colour may also be difficult to distinguish. The easiest colours for the elderly to see are usually reds, yellows and oranges.

The reduced visual sensitivity of old age is known as *presbyopia*. Yellowing and other changes of the lens lead to increasingly impaired visual acuity; seeing detail becomes very difficult and the lens loses some of its ability to *accommodate* to changes in distance vision so that it takes longer to see something distant after looking close to it. Some elderly people also develop specific eye disorders such as glaucoma, cataracts, macular degeneration and diabetic retinopathy. The changes in vision that occur can in themselves affect mobility, independence and confidence. Linked with failing hearing, they can have a profound effect upon the life of an older person (Erber, 2002).

iii) Touch

Touch sensitivity reduces with age making it increasingly difficult to manipulate items or to make fine adjustments (Erber, 2003) which can make it very difficult to insert, remove or operate a hearing aid.

3.3 THE PSYCHOLOGICAL AND SOCIAL EFFECTS OF AGEING

The brain has only a very limited capacity for repair following age-related changes, and some loss of function is almost inevitable.

Human memory is thought to consist of a short-term and a long-term memory. Short-term memory is seen as the ability to retain transient information for a few seconds. Working memory is related to short-term memory but extends beyond it. Hitch (2005) describes it as the:

'Ability to co-ordinate mental operations with transiently stored information during cognitive activities'.

Memory problems increase in the elderly, particularly with regard to short-term memory and with the ability to remember relatively recent experiences. Learning new information takes longer because of the reduced efficiency of neural transmission and poorer sensory input. The ability to retrieve stored information is also reduced. Long-term memory however seems to improve and events from many years ago may be remembered vividly.

Working memory decreases with age, possibly due to a decreasing ability to exclude unimportant detail. Encoding and retrieval of information that requires attention and concentration is limited by decreased working memory. An elderly person may, for example, have difficulty in remembering from the beginning of a story or message to the end of it, particularly when feeling under stress.

Memory problems may be increased by physical illness, medications or psychological conditions, such as depression. Memory performance tends to decline in depressed adults, whether or not they have impaired cognitive functioning. Self-esteem and self-confidence are often poor in old age, causing the person's motivation for learning and remembering new information also to be reduced.

Cognitive changes with age are in part due to reduced efficiency of nerve transmission in the brain causing slower and less efficient information processing. However, poor performance is also affected by other factors, such as slower motor ability and sensory deficits. For example, the elderly person has to give more attention and cognitive effort to comprehending sensory input and cannot therefore process new information as quickly.

Intelligence does not decline with age but older people require longer to complete tasks. Intelligence quotients (IQ) should not vary as IQ is calculated in comparison with the person's own age group.

Reaction time is reduced as old age increases (Birren and Fisher, 1995) and the more unexpected or the more complex the task, the slower is the reaction time. In some part this may be because the elderly tend to be more cautious and willing to sacrifice speed for accuracy. Sometimes they will not attempt something if they are uncertain (for example they have a tendency not to respond in audiometry, see *Figure 3.4*, until they are absolutely sure that they have heard a signal, which may result in thresholds appearing to be raised).

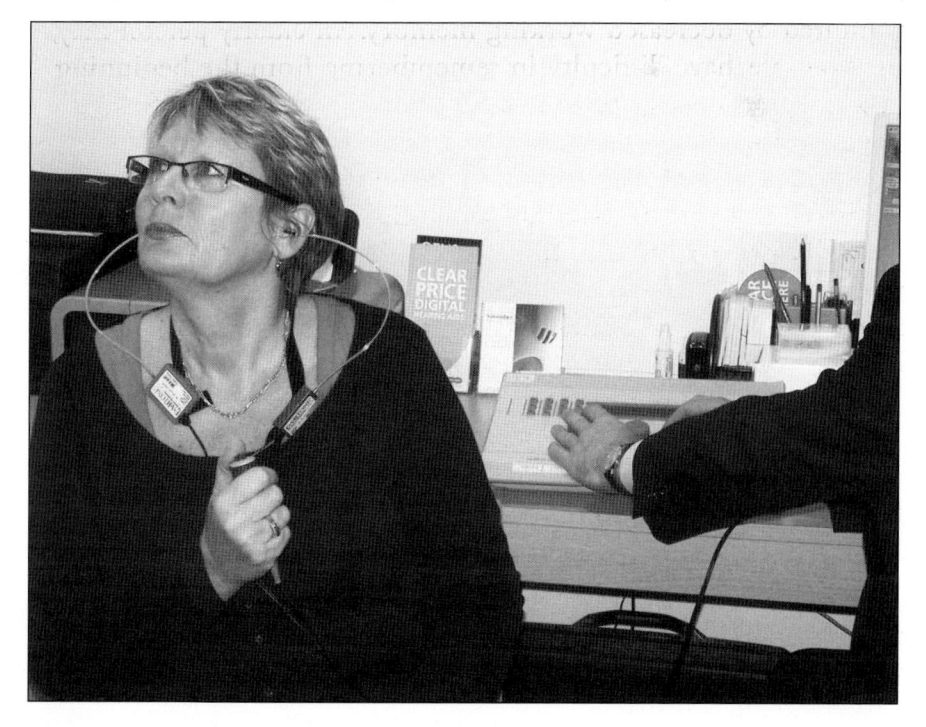

Figure 3.4 *An audiometric test (using ear inserts)*

Ageing is both a biological and a psychological process. Physical ageing impacts upon the individual and causes social and emotional difficulties as well as physical ones. The problems of ageing are real but cognitive decline is not inevitable. The way in which the person reacts to challenges and attempts to solve problems is as relevant as actual memory or learning ability. Older people often need more time to compensate for their slower physical and cognitive functioning but they can improve their functioning significantly with training and practice.

Old age brings with it life changes. Retirement is a large change that results in a reduction in income and the loss of work identity (Atchley, 2006) and may be considered as having a number of phases, although these do not necessarily follow in an orderly fashion, see *Table 3.1*.

The ageing process

Table 3.1 Phases of retirement (Atchley, 1974)

	Phases of retirement
1	*Pre-retirement* is the period in which retirement is anticipated.
2	*The retirement event* is generally a celebratory event.
3	*The honeymoon phase* follows, in which holidays and new hobbies are enjoyed.
4	*The rest and relaxation phase* is a short period in which the retiree enjoys respite from the obligations of work.
5	*The immediate retirement routine* is a readjustment to fill the days with useful activity.
6	*Disenchantment* is a period that may follow the honeymoon phase or which may be due to negative circumstances.
7	*Reorientation* is when realistic goals are set and new lifestyle decisions made to satisfy the goals.
8	*The retirement routine* is a stable period in which the new lifestyle is maintained.

Social roles change with retirement and the retired person may feel a sense of powerlessness and uselessness, especially if increased leisure time is not positively filled and structured. All change is stressful and older people sometimes resist change. Refusal of change is one method of maintaining control and, in order to accept change, they may need more explanation and more time to consider the proposed changes. Ageism prevails in our culture (despite changes to the law) and, in general, old people are stereotyped and discriminated against. In reality people retain their characteristics and are the same personalities as they were when they were younger. However, ageing brings major stresses and limited resources and the elderly are particularly vulnerable. Disease is common in old age and most of the elderly population (over 65) have at least one chronic disease, although in most it is not disabling.

3.4 COMMON CONDITIONS OF OLD AGE

3.4.1 Osteoporosis

This is a condition in which calcium is lost from the bones resulting in a decrease in bone mass. Gradually the spine may curve and the person loses height and develops a hump. The condition is caused by lack of both calcium and exercise. It is prevalent in elderly white women and may result in bone fractures, many of which are spontaneous, occurring without a fall.

3.4.2 Dementia

Dementia, sometimes referred to as senility, is a condition in which two or more of the faculties, such as language, memory and spatial abilities, are lost to a degree that interferes with daily life (Salama, 2008). Dementia is not a disease but a set of symptoms accompanying a disease such as Alzheimer's, Parkinson's or Huntingdon's disease. These diseases cause irreversible dementia. There are also cases of dementia that are reversible, such as those caused by depression, drugs or minor head injury. Most dementia, however, (56%) is due to Alzheimer's disease and almost half of elderly people over 85 have dementia.

Alzheimer's disease involves the formation of abnormal structures in the brain called *plaques* and *tangles* that accumulate and reduce the nerve cell connections. Initially they affect short-term memory but later they impair other intellectual and physical functions.

Parkinson's disease is concerned with the central nervous system and characterised by tremors (rhythmic shaking) in the extremities and muscle stiffness which causes slow movement, weak grasp and poor co-ordination.

Huntingdon's disease is a genetic condition, caused by a faulty gene on chromosome 4. The faulty gene damages nerve cells in the brain, which leads to gradual physical, mental and emotional changes. It is one of the most severe and frequent neurodegenerative diseases. The symptoms usually start between the ages of 30 and 50 but can start later. Symptoms include slight uncontrollable muscle movements, clumsiness, poor short-term memory, lack of concentration and changeable moods including depression, bad temper and aggression.

3.4.3 Hiatus hernia

This is protrusion of the stomach upwards through the opening of the oesophagus. The exact cause is unknown but it occurs when the muscle tissue surrounding the opening becomes weak, and the upper part of the stomach bulges up through the diaphragm into the chest cavity. Anything that places excessive pressure on the abdomen, e.g. persistent coughing, can contribute to a hernia. About 69% of people over 70 have this condition. Risk factors include:

- Aged over 50
- Obesity
- Smoking.

3.5 THEORIES OF AGEING

3.5.1 Introduction

Gerontology is the study of the ageing process and focuses on the normal processes of change in old age.

Ageing tends to be characterised by:

- Reduced adaptive ability
- Increased vulnerability to disease
- Physical and mental deterioration
- Increased mortality.

A *theory* is a collection of ideas or propositions intended to explain something and many theories have been proposed to explain ageing. However, there is no real consensus as to whether ageing is an unchangeable natural state (programmed theories) or a disease to be cured. Although we do not have a definitive answer as to why ageing occurs, it seems most likely that it is due to a number of causes acting at the same time. Whatever the cause or causes, our life expectancy is increasing and it seems therefore that the ageing process can at least be slowed.

3.5.2 Chemical damage (wear and tear theories)

The *wear and tear theories* of ageing suggest that the effects of ageing are caused by use. Over time the body cells will be worn out and become unable to function correctly. However, lack of use is perhaps more detrimental and gentle exercise can help the ageing body.

i) Rate of living theory

An early theory was the Rate of Living theory (Pearl, 1926) which was based on the observations by Max Rubner in 1908. The theory suggested that a fast basal metabolic rate corresponds to a short life span because the body will wear out quicker. This theory is now discredited.

ii) Reliability theory

Reliability theory is basically a statistical theory, originally designed for insurance purposes to work out probable failure rates. Mechanical failure is not unlike death. Death or failure can be regarded as an event for which the probability can be forecast. The reliability theory of ageing allows the prediction of age-related failure when the reliability of the body's components is known.

iii) Free radical theory

Harman (1956) produced a free radical theory of ageing. He suggested that free radicals (unstable high energy molecules produced by the body as by-products of normal energy production) damage other cells causing ageing.

iv) Auto-immune theory

This theory suggests that, with age, the immune system is less able to deal with foreign organisms and may increasingly attack its own body's tissues in error. Walford (1969) suggested that the normal process of ageing is genetically related to faulty immune processes.

v) The endocrine theory

The endocrine system controls the hormones that regulate many body processes. The endocrine theory of ageing suggests that the changes that cause the ageing process are brought about by hormones. Dysfunction of hormones and growth factors may play a critical role in ageing and cancer progression (Gilley et al, 2005). The neuro-endocrine control theory suggests that ageing is present to control the development and spread of cancer (Rodier et al, 2005). Since, in cancer, the cells can grow and multiply indefinitely, the limits set by ageing are important in controlling their spread.

3.5.3 Evolutionary (genetic) theories

Evolutionary or genetic theories of ageing suggest that:

i) Our natural lifespan is determined by our inherited genes and that this is therefore programmed at conception.
ii) Resources are invested in reproductive success even when this is at the expense of body maintenance later in life.

i) Programmed theory

Programmed theory suggests that a 'biological clock' or 'pacemaker' regulates ageing and that death is therefore programmed. The thymus gland (part of the immune system, see *Figure 3.5*) is sometimes suggested as being the biological clock. Weismann's programmed death theory (Goldsmith, 2004) suggested that ageing is an evolutionary trend in order that parents and their children do not have to compete for the same resources.

Hayflick (1965; 1996) found that human body cells are programmed to reproduce themselves a finite number of times. He took cells and let them reproduce until they eventually died. He found that most human cells die after about fifty doublings under ideal conditions. This fixed maximum capability is commonly known as 'the Hayflick limit'. However few cells are likely to reach their maximum due to physiological changes within the cell.

Telomeres are the DNA-protein complexes that cap chromosomal ends and promote chromosomal stability. Every time a cell divides its telomeres shorten. Thus the length of the telomeres can act as a biomarker of a cell's biological age. When the telomeres reach a critically short length, the cell stops dividing. Telomere length is significantly shortened by psychological stress (Epel et al, 2004), which may be related to the early onset of age-related diseases.

Telomerase is a cellular enzyme that synthesises and preserves telomeres and which can reset the number of times a cell can multiply (Harley, 1992; Bodnar et al, 1998). Hormones are crucially involved in regulating telomerase activity (Bayne and Liu, 2005). In theory at least, the telomerase gene could prolong life significantly (Betts and Madan, 2008; Aubert and Lansdorp, 2008; Haussmann and Mauck, 2008) by lengthening the telomere. It seems that the telomeres are the biological clock and that the enzyme telomerase may be able to rewind the clock to increase life span. Telomerase is claimed to be potentially important for the treatment of cancer and age-related disease (Kim et al, 1994, 2002).

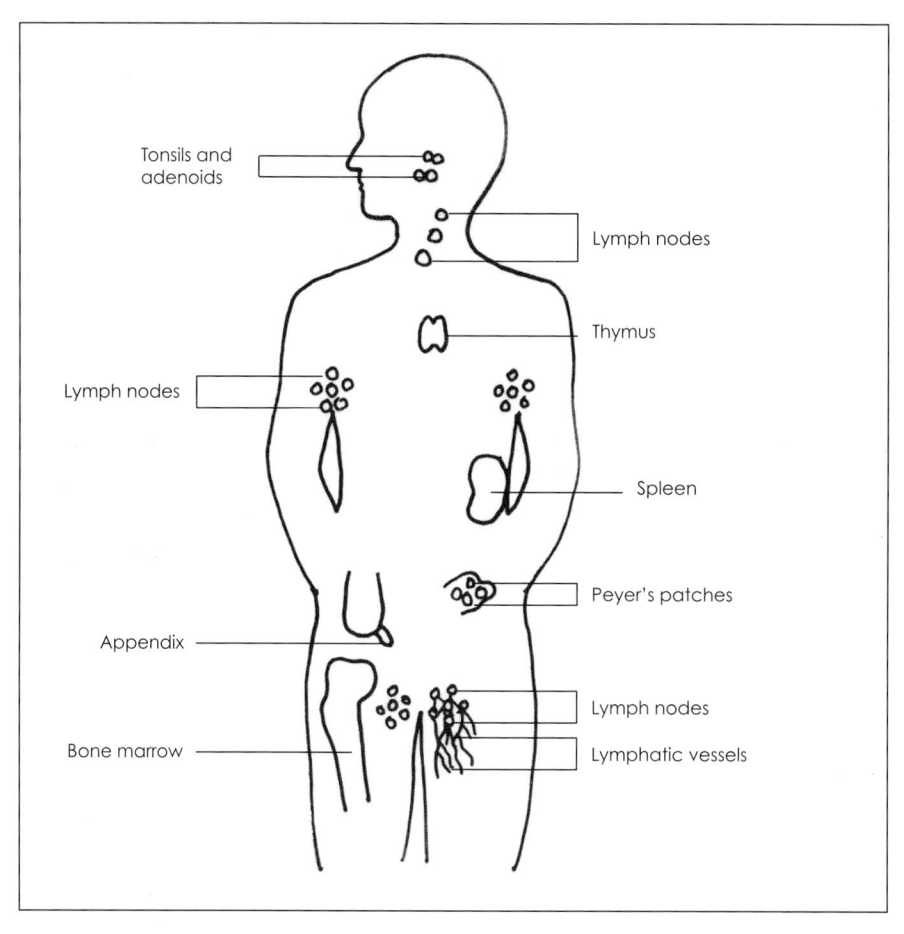

Figure 3.5 *The immune system (Reproduced with kind permission of Anglia Distance Learning Ltd)*

ii) The mutation accumulation theory

Haldane (1941) theorised that Huntington's disease remained in the population and was not eliminated by natural selection because the onset of the disease normally occurs around the age of 45, which is after the adult's reproductive period has ended. The theory views ageing as 'little more than a dustbin of late acting gene mutations... which could not be eliminated by natural selection' (Lane, 2005). Haldane made the assumption that, in ancient times, few people survived beyond the age of 45. The contribution of these few older people to the next generation was relatively small and therefore such late-acting mutations were relatively unimportant. A mutation affecting younger people would be much more likely to be affected by natural selection.

Medawar (1952) formalised this observation into the mutation accumulation theory of ageing. The theory states that ageing results from harmful mutations that occur relatively late in life. A genetic change late in life will be relatively unimportant and natural selection will not act against late mutations. These harmful mutations can therefore accumulate and eventually cause death.

Others developed this theory further and their ideas form the basis of our current understanding of evolutionary influence on ageing. Williams (1957), for example, published a complementary theory based on the notion that one gene will affect a variety of different traits and that, if a gene will improve fitness early on, it will be favoured by evolution – even though it may be at the expense of reduced fitness later on in life. The theory was further extended (Kirkwood, 1991) by emphasizing that evolution has led to an optimum balance between metabolic energy for reproduction versus that required for the maintenance of the body's cells.

3.5.4 Summary

Normal ageing involves a number of physical, sensory and psychological changes. Physical changes include atrophy of muscles and bones, together with hormonal changes. Older people also have more chronic disease than younger adults but these conditions are not usually disabling.

No part of the hearing system is impervious to changes that occur with age but only changes to the inner ear have any real impact on hearing sensitivity. Hearing loss is typically a gradual loss affecting mainly the high frequencies. Speech understanding may be poorer than the audiogram would suggest due to central auditory problems.

Visual acuity decreases gradually from about the age of forty and normal vision is rare after the age of sixty. Wounds heal more slowly. Sense of touch starts to dull and this can make handling hearing aids difficult. Psychological changes include a reduction in working memory and an inability to exclude background noise and other extraneous information. The elderly need more time to succeed in learning tasks.

Theories of ageing seek to explain the process. These theories fall into two groups, genetic or environmental theories and chemical damage or wear and tear theories. It is most likely that the ageing process is in fact due to a number of causes acting at the same time.

Chapter 4
Beginning the Rehabilitation Process

4.1 THE REHABILITATION PROCESS

The rehabilitation process starts from the first contact with a client and may well include information obtained prior to meeting in person. The process can be broken down into five main stages (see *Figure 4.1*), which are:

1. *Assessment*: Information is gathered from the client (and their companion if one is present), most commonly using an interview technique. The client's needs and problems are determined. Questionnaires can be helpful in obtaining a list of problem areas that can also form the basis for quantitative evaluation of hearing aid benefit at stage 4. The audiologist will use audiometric tests to obtain information regarding hearing status, which will include pure tone thresholds and possibly further tests, for example speech recognition. Other useful information such as visual acuity, mental function, attitude and manual dexterity should also be noted.
2. *Decision-making*: This is where the information from stage 1 is reviewed and acted upon in decisions regarding amplification and a rehabilitation plan. Goals are set.
3. *Remediation*: The client is guided so they can make informed choices. Hearing aids are chosen and fitted. Tactics are taught. Counselling and communication

training are undertaken. Assistive devices are introduced when appropriate.
4. *Evaluation*: The success of the rehabilitation programme is evaluated and modifications are made and further counselling, etc. undertaken as required.
5. *On-going rehabilitation*: The audiologist continues to be available to the client when needed. Further help is particularly likely to be sought when hearing changes are noted.

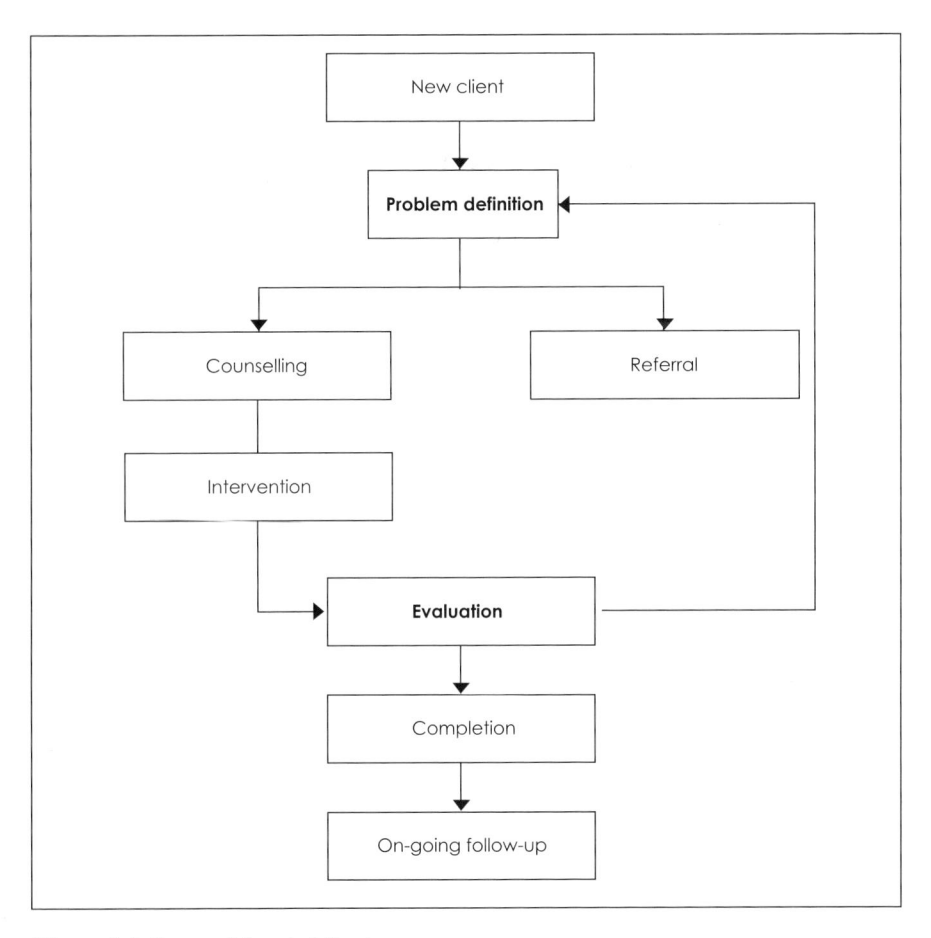

```
                    ┌─────────────┐
                    │ New client  │
                    └──────┬──────┘
                           ▼
                 ┌───────────────────┐
              ┌─▶│ Problem definition│◀──┐
              │  └─────────┬─────────┘   │
              │       ┌────┴────┐        │
              │       ▼         ▼        │
              │  ┌─────────┐ ┌────────┐  │
              │  │Counselling│ │Referral│  │
              │  └────┬────┘ └────────┘  │
              │       ▼                  │
              │  ┌──────────┐            │
              │  │Intervention│           │
              │  └────┬─────┘            │
              │       ▼                  │
              │  ┌──────────┐            │
              └─▶│Evaluation│────────────┘
                 └────┬─────┘
                      ▼
                 ┌──────────┐
                 │Completion│
                 └────┬─────┘
                      ▼
              ┌────────────────┐
              │On-going follow-up│
              └────────────────┘
```

Figure 4.1 Stages of the rehabilitative process

4.2 ASSESSMENT AND DECISION-MAKING IN THE INITIAL CONSULTATION

4.2.1 The case history

The more information that can be gleaned at the initial consultation, the more appropriate the individual rehabilitation plan is likely to be. Ideally a partner or close family member should accompany the client to the first meeting with the audiologist as this person will be able to support the client and may also provide useful information in addition to (and sometimes conflicting with!) that provided by the client.

It is important to consider all the factors that may be relevant, including whether the client actually accepts that they have a hearing disability. If the client has been persuaded by others to seek help and has not come under their own initiative, it is quite likely that they have not yet accepted their hearing loss. Some clients really are unaware that they have a problem but it is much more usual to find clients who may be aware but who are too afraid or embarrassed to admit to it. The client's attitude to intervention is critical to the success of the process and some clients will be motivated whilst others will remain negative and may be very reluctant to use hearing aids.

The case history is usually the first part of the assessment process and it is during the case history that the audiologist will seek to find possible answers for the cause of hearing loss and information concerning other medical conditions, age, personality and lifestyle. Sufficient accurate information is essential as some clinical decisions may be based on the case history. It also allows the audiologist to get to know the client and to discover what they expect from the consultation and what their attitude is to using hearing aids. A useful list of what the client sees as their problem areas can be obtained through questions such as "What effect does your hearing loss have on your life?" When answering the client should be encouraged to list all the effects that they can. Alternatively, standard questionnaires can be used and these can also help to quantify improvement after the hearing aid has been fitted.

All new hearing aid users require some degree of counselling but extra counselling will be needed if, for example, their expectations are unrealistic, they are not prepared to use hearing aids or they are very self-conscious about wearing aids. Education about the hearing loss and what to expect from hearing aids will often help in reaching understanding and acceptance. Clients must be encouraged to work through any negativity and grief in order that they may come to terms with their hearing loss because a positive attitude (or at least a willingness to try) is important in achieving success. The audiologist's role includes supporting the client psychologically as well as physically and this supportive role runs throughout the rehabilitative process, see *Table 4.1*.

Table 4.1 Tasks involved in the audiologist's initial consultation (based on Silverman et al, 1998)

	Tasks involved in the initial consultation
1	*Initiate the consultation*: Greet the client, establish initial rapport and identify the reason(s) for the consultation.
2	*Gather information*: Explain that notes will be taken. Explore the problem(s), understand the client's perspective and provide structure to the consultation.
3	*Build a relationship*: Develop rapport. Empower the client to express their ideas, concerns and expectations, to ask questions and to seek clarification.
4	*Explain and plan*: Provide appropriate high quality information, use terms the client will understand. Share decision-making.
5	*Close the consultation*: Clarify and summarise to enhance understanding and adherence to the rehabilitation programme.

4.2.2 Assessment procedures

All procedures and their rationale should be described to the client and their partner or family member prior to proceeding. Every part of the consultation process can help address the client's attitude, needs and education as well as providing the direct information required by the audiologist.

In most instances a hearing test will be carried out, see *Figure 4.2*. After the test, the results should be carefully explained. The client (and the person accompanying them) usually has little understanding of hearing loss and an appropriate explanation of their hearing test results and the effect of their hearing loss will often lead to the client recognising the problem as their own.

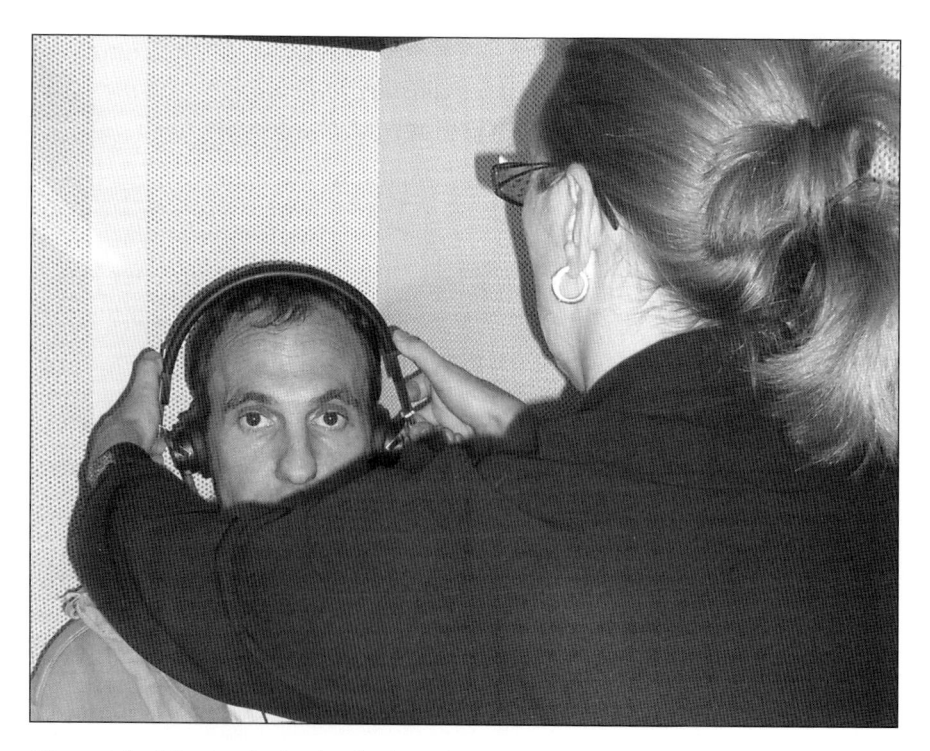

Figure 4.2 *Adjusting the headset for the audiometric test*

The audiogram, see *Figure 4.3*, can be explained as a chart or graph showing the hearing test results. It is often helpful to indicate on the audiogram the area of normal hearing and also to divide the audiogram to illustrate low frequencies and high frequencies. By now the audiologist will know the client's background and therefore should be able to pitch the explanation at an appropriate level, avoiding unfamiliar terminology. The explanation will normally start with the axes of the graph, for example:

> Across the bottom, the graph shows the tones you heard. **(Indicate an imaginary split down the graph at 1kHz)**. These are the low tones and these are the high tones.
>
> Down the side of the graph it shows how loud the sounds were. This line **(0dBHL)** is what we consider to be normal hearing, although we don't usually expect anyone to have too much difficulty if their hearing is between here and here **(-10 to 20dBHL area)**.
>
> This symbol **(0)** is for your right ear and this **(X)** is for your left. The 0s and Xs on the graph show the level of sound you can **just** hear...
>
> The frequencies might also be compared to a piano keyboard where the keys must be struck harder in the high frequencies (pitches) to hear them.

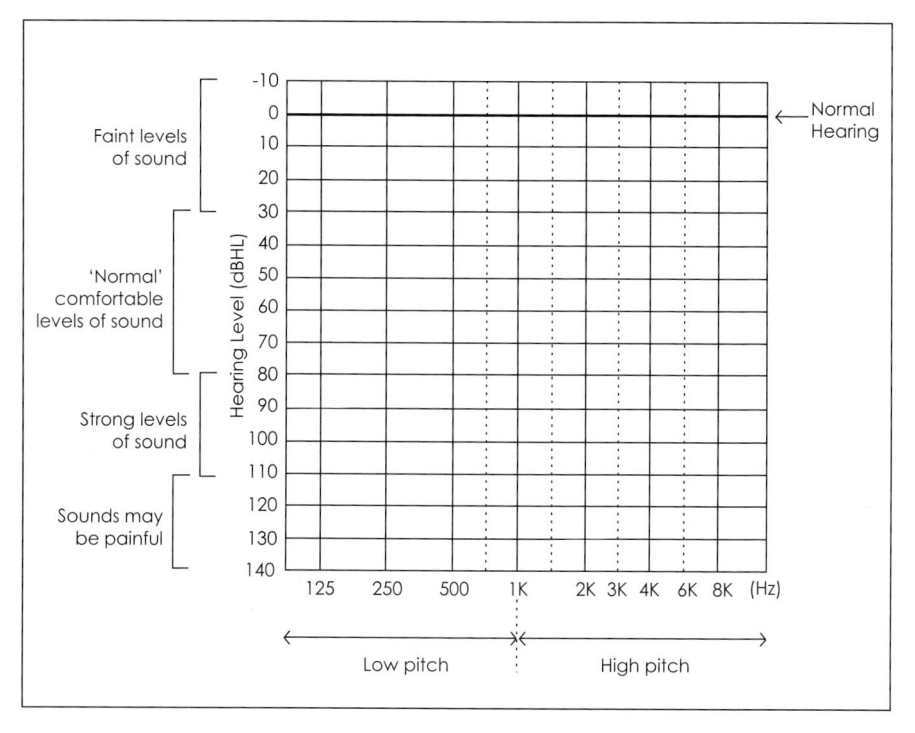

Figure 4.3 An audiogram explained

High frequency hearing is usually affected most and it can be explained that this affects the clarity of speech rather than the volume. If recorded speech to simulate hearing loss is not available, it may help to use written phrases or sentences with first the consonants and then the vowels missing to demonstrate this, see *Figure 4.4*. Situations that the client finds particularly difficult can be related to the hearing loss and also to the effects of noise.

```
-a- - / a - - / - i - -  / - e - - / u - / - - e / - i - - .
J – c k / - n d / J - l l / w – n t / - p / t h - / h – l l.
```

Figure 4.4 *A sentence written without consonants and then without vowels*

Bone conduction results also need to be pointed out with an explanation of where the problem appears to lie and whether or not it is likely to be permanent or progressive. The client should be asked if they have any questions and these should be answered honestly. If medical or surgical intervention to restore the hearing is inappropriate, as is usually the case, hearing aids may provide the best option and the audiologist needs to combine emotional support with giving practical advice on the choice of hearing aids.

4.2.3 Hearing aid choice

Clients usually like to have choice, but too wide a range of aids can be confusing. The client may have reasons to prefer certain types of aid (for example wanting inconspicuous aids) but by listening to their needs the audiologist will usually be able to introduce a small range (about three) of suitable hearing aids. Sometimes the client wants an inappropriate type of aid (perhaps, for example, someone with a severe manipulation problem might want a very small aid that they cannot physically manage) but if enough time is spent explaining and demonstrating the advantages and disadvantages of the different options, the audiologist will usually be able to assist the client in coming to an appropriate choice.

It is important to tell the client what it may be like to hear through a hearing aid. In particular, they need to know in advance that a hearing aid does not restore natural hearing, that their own voice will sound strange and that they will need to get used to sounds again, particularly if they have not heard well for some time. Allowing the client to wear appropriately set aids in the quiet test room, using temporary ear fittings, is often a positive experience and one that gives the audiologist the chance to discuss how the aid sounds to the client, and the programme of wearing that is suggested, whilst they become accustomed to amplification. If two aids are being advised, two aids should be fitted for demonstration. They should be fitted before they are switched on so that feedback is avoided and ideally they should be left in place throughout the remainder of the consultation. If possible, the aids should not be fine-tuned but, unless the aids are of the 'instant fit' type, the client should understand that they are intended only to give them an idea of what amplification is like and that the aids they will have will not sound exactly the same.

Free field speech tests without and then with the hearing aids can be very helpful in demonstrating benefit and, similarly, it can be helpful to have the partner or family member converse with the client to illustrate their improved listening ability. However, if the client has good speech understanding in quiet conditions whilst unaided, such demonstrations are likely to be *un*helpful and should be avoided, as little or no improvement may be shown in the test room situation!

The client should be allowed to handle demonstration or dummy aids similar to those they will have. Handling the aids and their controls will help them to become more confident, see *Figure 4.5*. When they have made their decision, ear impressions will be taken as appropriate and paper work completed. The fitting appointment (or follow up for instantly fitted aids) should be arranged and the client should be advised or reminded of what will happen next, making sure that they fully understand.

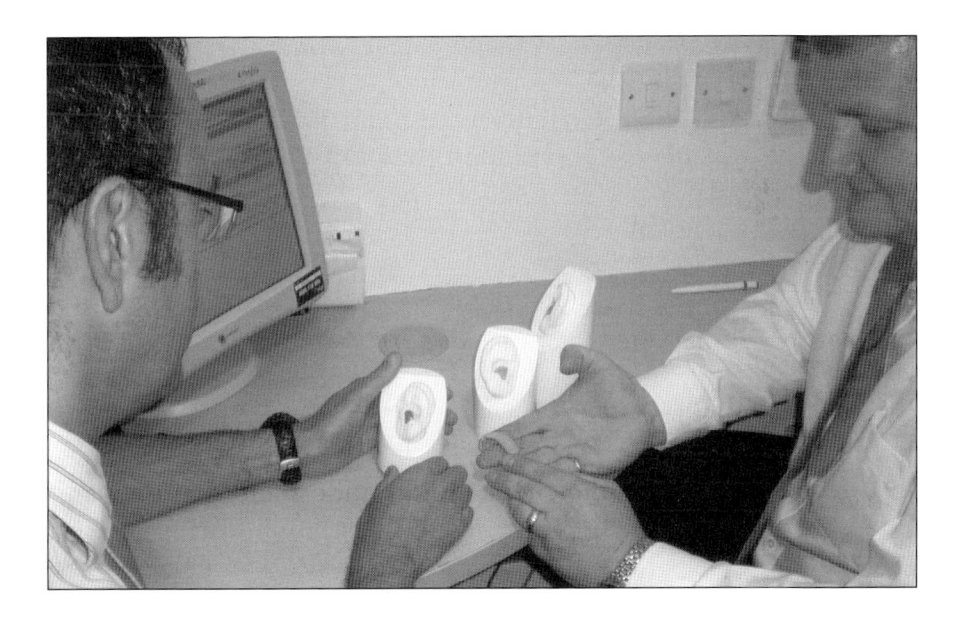

Figure 4.5 A client making the aid choice

At the fitting appointment, the client will be instructed on how to insert and remove the aids, how to maintain them and when and how to use them. They can practice putting the aids in place and also fitting and removing batteries. The client (or a carer) must be able to do these successfully or they will not be able to manage the aids. They can also be given tips on how the listening environment may be improved and a further appointment should be made to assess their progress and address any future problems. Rehabilitation does not stop at the first appointment and should continue through the hearing aid fitting, the follow up appointment, in repair sessions and whenever there is a change in circumstances.

4.3 COMMUNICATION SKILLS FOR THE AUDIOLOGIST

4.3.1 Interaction skills

The audiologist's interaction with the client can help or hinder their decision-making. Communication between client and audiologist must be as effective as possible so that the client will heed the advice they are given, make an appropriate choice and be able to use and maintain the aids well.

If a client does not readily express their concerns, needs and expectations, the audiologist requires the communication skills to discover them. It is only by encouraging the client to talk about their problems that the audiologist can hope to meet the client's needs. The audiologist should listen actively, use appropriate questioning techniques and clarify and summarise. In this way they can gather information and give advice and instruction.

4.3.2 Active listening

Active listening means paying full attention and appearing to be interested. Full attention takes concentration and effort and involves attending to both verbal and non-verbal communication. Verbal cues are speech features other than words, for example volume and pitch. Non-verbal cues are non-speech features, for example facial expression and gesture. It is not only what the client is saying that is important; their tone of voice, facial expression, gestures and eye contact, etc. can also impart useful information about their feelings. For instance someone who is:

- Angry or excited: will often speak quickly.
- Stressed: will often fidget.
- Nervous: may falter over their words.

Clients are only likely to communicate well with the audiologist if they believe the audiologist is interested in them. Interest can be shown by making appropriate facial expressions, gestures (e.g. nodding), short comments or encouraging noises (e.g. 'mm' or 'uh huh') and allowing the client time to respond. Reflecting on what has been said by repeating back the last few words of a salient point can also demonstrate active listening and may be used to clarify what has been said. In general, it is good to appear confident and open and this may be helped by:

- Adopting a confident, relaxed posture to give a good impression and put the client at ease.
- Smiling, particularly on meeting, to make the audiologist appear more approachable.
- Maintaining appropriate eye contact to show interest and build trust. Eye contact is very important but continuous eye contact or staring may appear threatening and unsettling.
- Keeping hands away from the face, as this can detract attention from the conversation.
- Not folding the arms, as this can give the appearance of impatience.
- Not fidgeting, as this can give the appearance of a lack of interest.

4.3.3 Questioning techniques

To obtain information from the client the audiologist will ask questions which may be either open or closed. Closed questions can be answered briefly, usually by yes or no. They elicit only the information requested and usually nothing more. They can be useful in gathering or checking straightforward information and for putting the client at ease but for expansion of the subject the questions used should be open and will often be of the 'Why?' or 'How?' type. A more descriptive answer may also be gained by being direct and asking the client to expand on the subject. Some simple examples of open and closed questions are given in *Table 4.2*. Once a question has been asked the client must be allowed time to answer. It is important not to cut the client off in mid-flow as this will not help achieve good rapport. However there are helpful cues to when a person has finished speaking, which should be noted, for example leaving a longer gap and tending to look up when finishing speaking.

Table 4.2 Examples of open and closed questions

Closed	Open
Do you like this aid?	How do you feel about this aid?
Is it difficult to hear in a crowd?	What sort of situations do you find difficult?
Where does it hurt?	How would you describe it?
Do you think you need hearing aids?	Why do you think your daughter says you have difficulty in hearing?
What work do you do?	Can you tell me a little about the work you do?

4.4 REFLECTIVE PRACTICE

The Kolb learning cycle considers learning as experiential, that is learning comes through experience. Kolb (1984) suggested that ideas are not fixed but can be modified through previous experience.

The learning cycle, *Figure 4.6*, provides a useful descriptive model of the adult learning process, consisting of four stages:

1. *Concrete Experience*: direct practical experience (doing).
2. *Reflective Observation*: generalising from the experience (reviewing).
3. *Abstract Conceptualisation*: generating ideas for modification and improvement (learning).
4. *Active Experimentation*: leading to a modified concrete experience (applying).

Reflective observation allows critical self-analysis of decision making processes and highlights problems and gaps in knowledge and skill, which should then lead onto a change in behaviour (learning). However, it is not only the client who should be learning from their experiences. Reflection is an important skill for the professional audiologist to develop and use. Reflective practice (stage 2) involves analysing or evaluating experiences, applying theory to practice, making generalisations, validating effective practice or constructing different approaches. Reflective practice results in personal and professional development through critical thinking and is a core element in developing professional expertise (Schon, 1983; Ghaye et al, 1996; Tate and Sills, 2004).

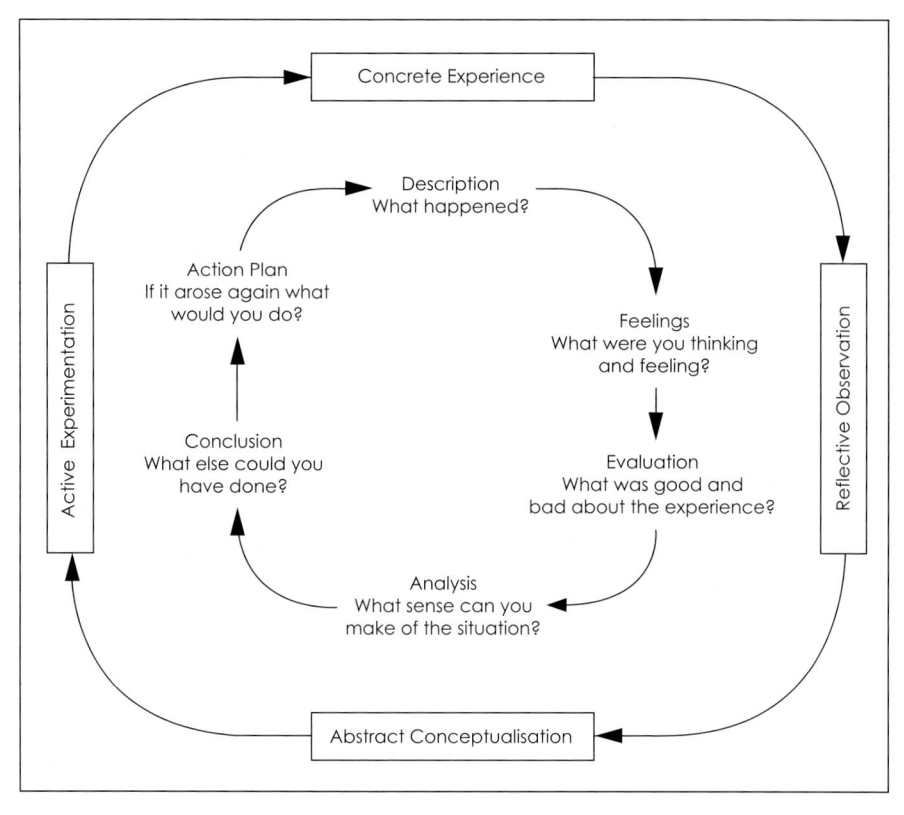

Figure 4.6 An experiential learning cycle (based on the Kolb learning cycle (1984) and the reflective cycle of Gibbs, 1988)

Chapter 5
Amplification

5.1 MODERN HEARING AIDS

5.1.1 The purpose of hearing aids

Hearing aids are instruments that are intended to enable hearing impaired people to obtain the maximum benefit from their residual hearing. Hearing aids are therefore generally required to provide:

- Optimum speech intelligibility
- Maximum useful information from other sounds
- Maximum comfort and sound quality
- Minimum distortion and interference from unwanted background noise.

Hearing aids are least useful in noisy situations and user satisfaction is strongly correlated with the number of listening situations in which the user perceives benefit (Kochkin, 2002).

5.1.2 Hearing aid types

Most hearing aid types, see *Figure 5.1*, utilise the normal air conduction route, via the outer and middle ear. Air conduction (normal) hearing aids are like a miniature public address system that is worn either behind or in the ear. Sound waves strike the microphone of the hearing aid and are converted to electrical signals, which are processed (including being amplified), converted back to sound and delivered to the ear. A small number of hearing aids send the sound directly to the cochlea by bone conduction. Bone conduction hearing aids use a vibrating receiver placed on the mastoid process, see *Figure 5.2*, which transmits vibrations to the cochlea through the bones of the skull. This type of hearing aid is used in some cases of conductive hearing loss, generally when it would not be advisable to block the ear canal. Bone conduction aids are less flexible in terms of style and sound processing and not suited to sensorineural hearing losses.

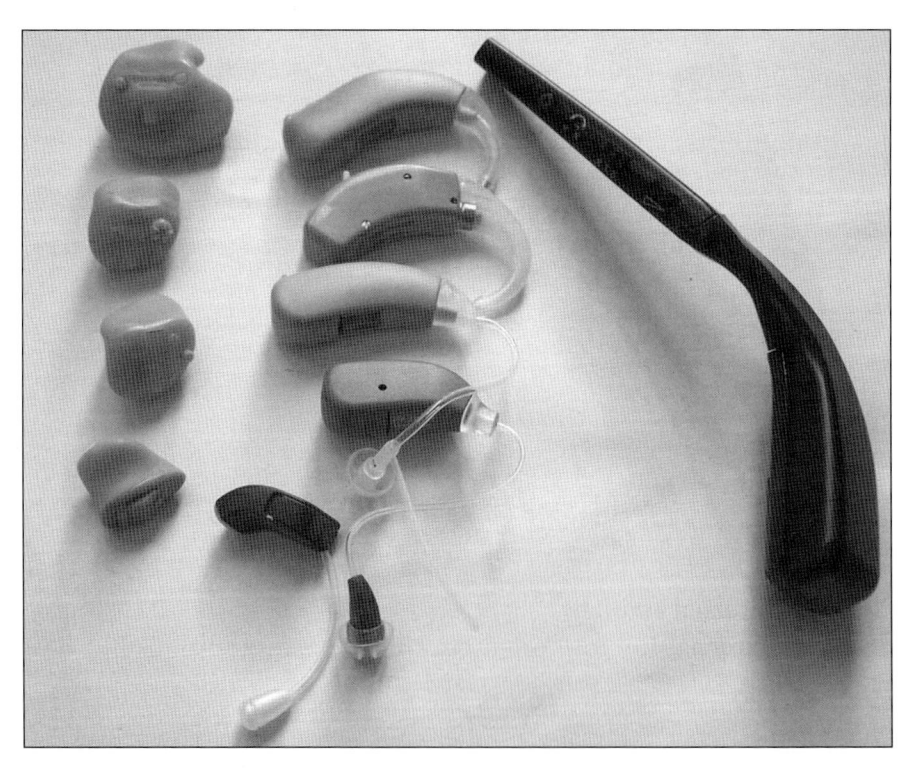

Figure 5.1 *Hearing aid types (Left to Right: In the ear; Behind the ear; Bone conduction spectacles – arm only shown)*

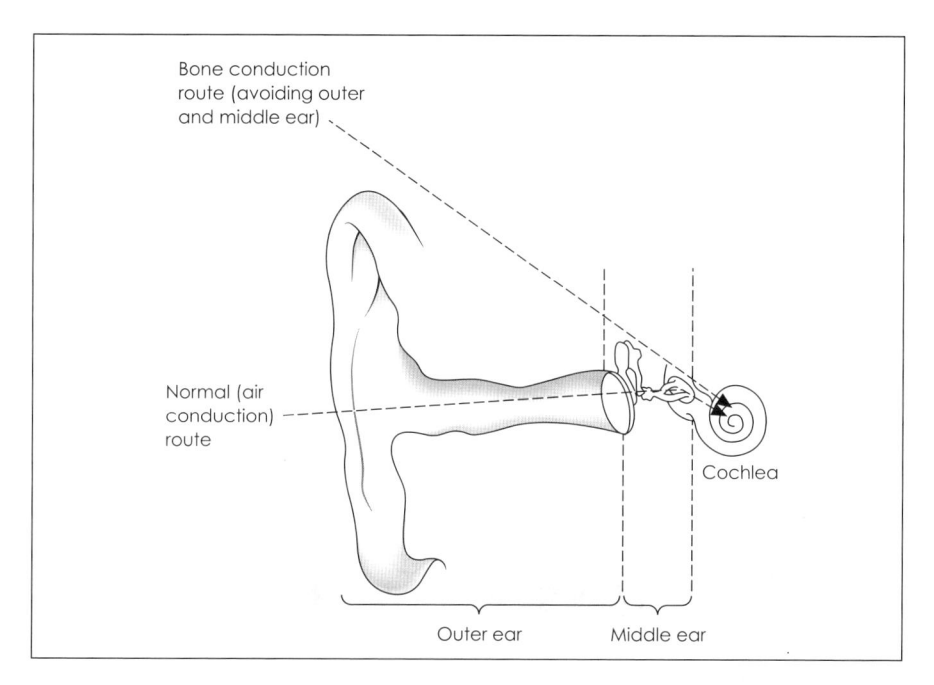

Figure 5.2 *Bone conduction and air conduction routes*

5.1.3 Cochlear implants

A cochlear implant is a special type of hearing aid, see *Figure 5.3*, which bypasses the hair cells of the cochlea and directly stimulates the auditory nerve. The device is not fully implanted as the name would suggest but consists of:

- An internal implant
- An external microphone, speech processor and transmitting coil.

Sounds enter the microphone and passes to the speech processing unit, where digital signal processing occurs. Cochlear implants are individually programmed and the results are saved as a 'map'. The processed signal is passed to the transmitting coil and transmitted to an internal receiver. The signal is sent from the receiver to an electrode array, which has been placed surgically in the cochlea. The electrodes that receive the signal 'fire' and send an electrical signal up the auditory nerve to the brain. The processed electrical signal is interpreted by the brain and is heard as mechanical-sounding speech.

Amplification

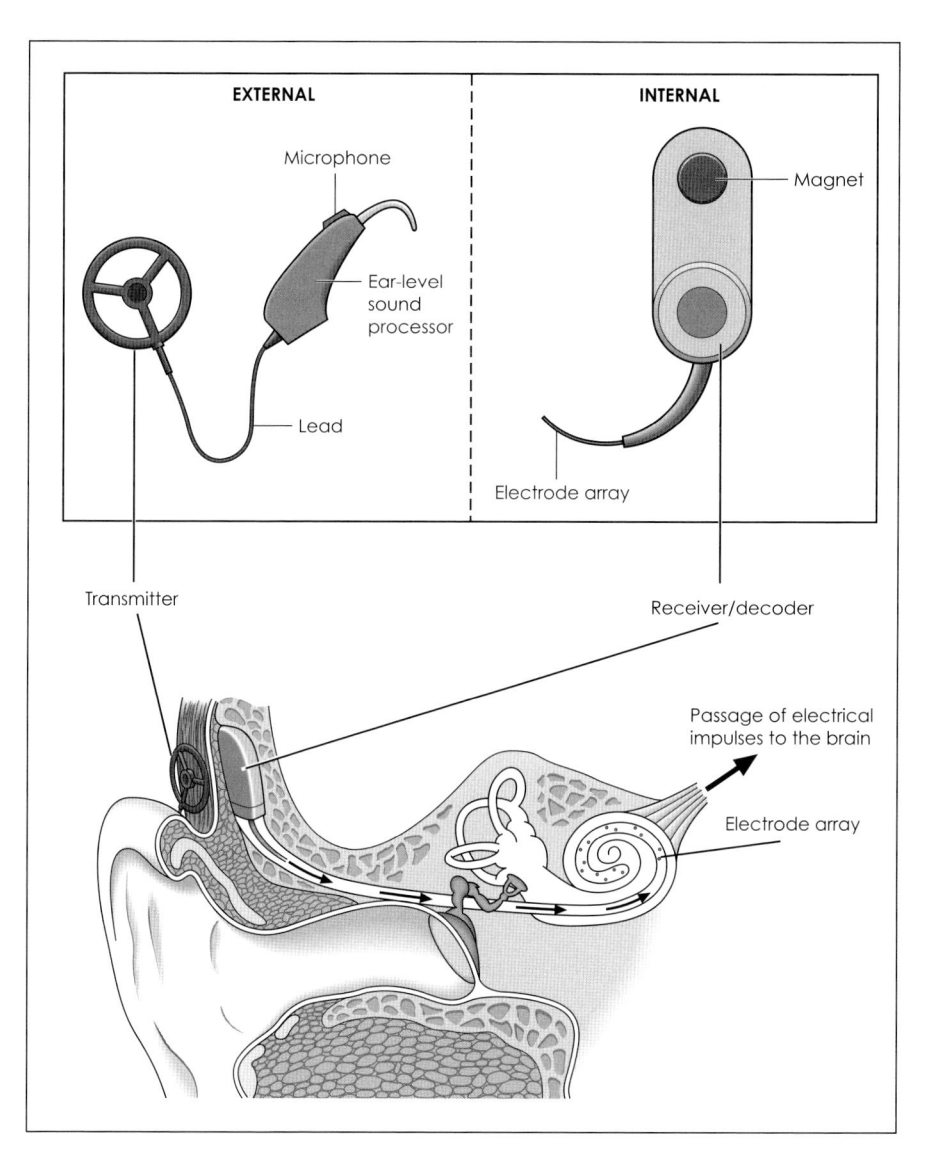

Figure 5.3 A cochlear implant

Almost all implants are multichannel and consist of a number of electrodes (usually twenty or more) which are placed at intervals along the length of the array. Frequency information is recognised according to the place along the cochlea at which the nerve is stimulated. Thus information regarding frequency can be maintained by stimulating the appropriate electrodes.

Cochlear implants are used where only limited benefit is obtained from conventional hearing aids, usually due to bilateral severe to profound sensorineural deafness. The degree of success depends on a number of variables, for example:

- Motivation
- Onset of deafness
- Length of auditory deprivation before fitting
- Health of the auditory nerve.

People with acquired deafness are generally very successful candidates for implantation as their experience of speech and language allows them to perform well. Children who are born deaf may also be considered for cochlear implants, usually at an early age. Cochlear implants may be used binaurally, monaurally or in conjunction with a hearing aid in the non-implanted ear. Cochlear implants often lead to great positive benefits such as improved confidence and general quality of life but they do not restore normal hearing and the degree of benefit varies between individuals. The implantation programme always involves extensive rehabilitation.

5.2 HEARING AID PROCESSING

Conventional hearing aids may use analogue or digital signal processing but most aids are now digital and, since the introduction of digital signal processing, they have become

Amplification

increasingly sophisticated. All hearing aids consist of a microphone, an amplifying device, a power source, user controls and a 'receiver' or loudspeaker. The processing strategy used (analogue or digital) does not affect the outer appearance of the aid.

Digital hearing aids convert the sound signal into a digital or numeric signal because this can be easily manipulated. The digital signal can be analysed in a great variety of ways, for example speech can be separated from noise, feedback can be separated from the original sound signal, and individual characteristics can be independently processed. Options that are available to improve the listening experience include:

- *Directional microphones* are designed to improve speech audibility in noisy situations. Conventional microphones are omni directional, which means they accept sound from all directions. A directional microphone suppresses sound from certain directions. Early directional microphones consisted of one microphone with two sound entry points or 'ports'. A time delay network was inserted in the rear sound path, such that background noise would reach the microphone from both ports at the same time. In this way background noise would be cancelled out, see *Figure 5.4*. Many hearing aids now have two or more microphones rather than having two ports into one microphone. The distance between the separate microphones creates small differences in the sound received by each, so that unwanted sound can be cancelled out or reduced. However, having two microphones also allows switching between omni directional and directional modes according to the listening situation.

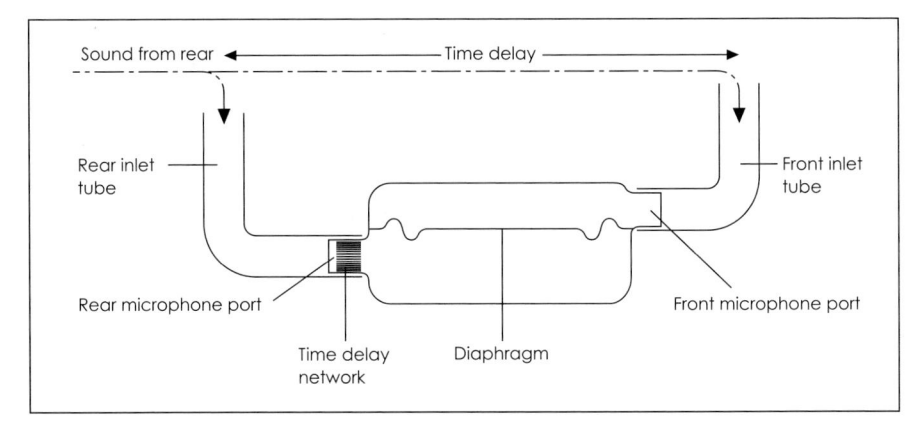

Figure 5.4 An early directional microphone (Reproduced with kind permission of Maltby, 2002)

- *Compression* automatically reduces the gain or amplification as the volume or intensity of the sound input increases. Compression is appropriate with sensorineural hearing loss but the hearing loss and the noise type will dictate the compression strategy to be used. *Compression limiting* does not affect the input until near the maximum output when, without causing noticeable distortion, it keeps the sound from reaching an uncomfortable level. *Wide dynamic range compression* varies the level of gain according to the input. With sensorineural loss, the ability to hear quiet sounds is reduced but the ability to tolerate loud sounds does not increase and may also reduce. This means that the difference between the individual's hearing threshold and their uncomfortable loudness level (i.e. their dynamic range, see *Figure 5.5*) is decreased. Wide dynamic range compression attempts to restore the sensation of normal loudness growth by providing mild gain for soft inputs and increasingly less gain for higher input levels. As a result quiet sounds are amplified so that they become audible, speech intensities are increased to a comfortable level and loud sounds are restricted to a tolerable level. In many hearing aids the compression strategy will vary across the frequency range, which is appropriate because the hearing loss tends to vary across the frequency range and also not all sounds contain the same amount of energy in the different frequency regions.

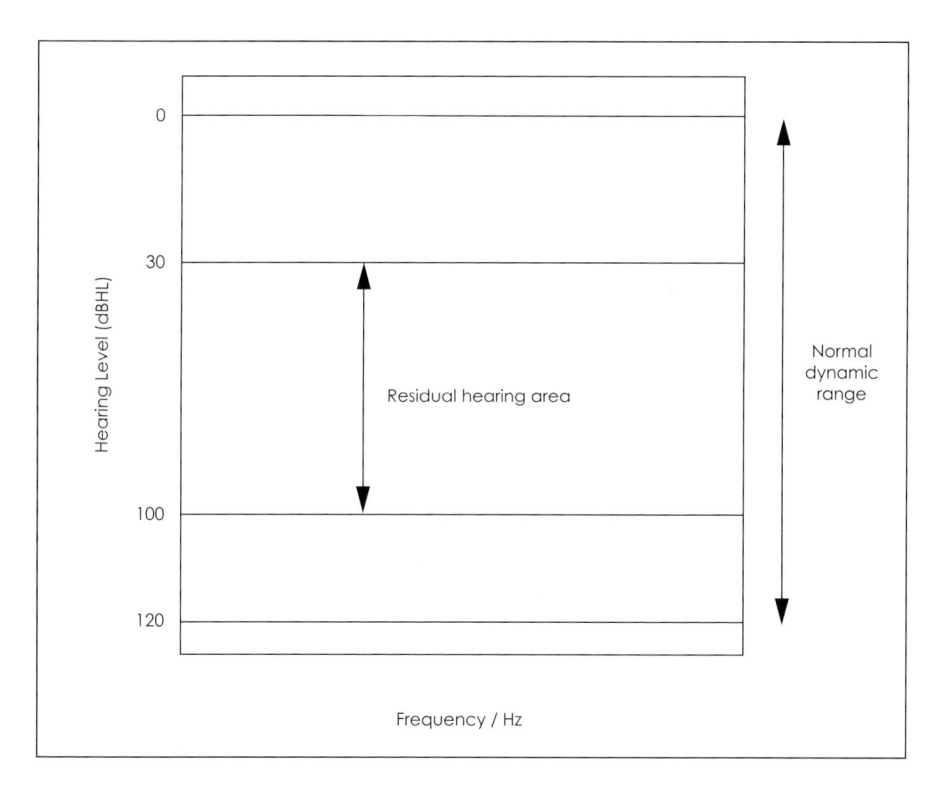

Figure 5.5 Residual hearing area or 'dynamic range' (Reproduced with kind permission of Maltby, 2002)

- *Noise reduction* systems are applied to reduce the gain (amplification) when noise is detected. The signal in the hearing aid is separated into independently manipulated frequency bands so the gain is only reduced where necessary and the rest of the signal is unchanged.
- *Multiple programmes* allow the user to switch between two or more programmes to suit their environment. Each programme will be set appropriately for a particular listening situation, for example for quiet situations, noisy situations and music. Some hearing aids can analyse the acoustic environment and classify it into the appropriate situation automatically.
- *Feedback control systems* act to reduce or cancel feedback (whistling) from the hearing aid. Feedback occurs when sound leaks from the ear back to the microphone of the aid. Feedback control systems may reduce the gain in the frequency region which is causing the feedback, use feedback cancellation where the feedback is cancelled by an equal and opposite (out of phase) sound signal or alter the frequency of a narrow band of the sound output so that it varies slightly from the input.
- 'True' binaural (as opposed to bilateral, which is also called binaural) systems, see *Figure 5.6*, use two hearing aids that are able to 'talk' to each other via a wireless link. The two aids act as a single binaural system (a pair) using common noise management and directional microphone settings. Using two aids working together improves localisation and means that the user can control both aids simultaneously, for example when the programme is changed.

Amplification

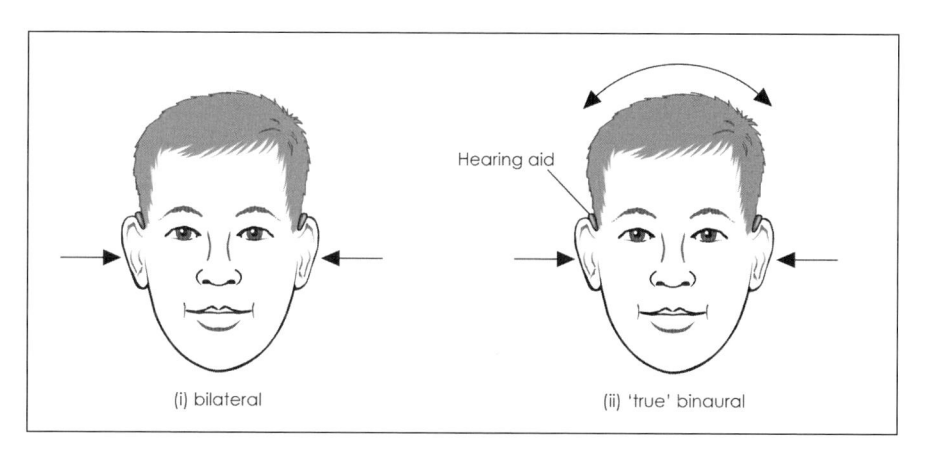

Figure 5.6 Bilateral and 'true' binaural systems

5.3 TEACHING HEARING AID MANAGEMENT

5.3.1 Introduction

Formal instruction in hearing aid management, including cleaning and maintenance, insertion and removal, battery replacement and acclimatisation, is needed if the aids are to be used and maintained correctly. The user will only benefit from their hearing aids if they are shown how to use them to best advantage and also helped to understand their limitations.

5.3.2 The first-time hearing aid user

The audiologist should ensure that the aids fit comfortably in the client's ears and set the controls to provide optimum sound quality and speech discrimination. The new hearing aid user then needs to learn how to position the aid in the ear, fit batteries, use the volume control, etc. and how to approach using the hearing aid in order to get the best out of it.

If possible, the client should be shown the controls on another aid of the same type. Any user controls should be explained and the battery type and how to replace one should be discussed in detail. The client needs to know how long the battery is likely to last, when it should be changed and how to insert and remove one.

The client will need to be shown how to fit the hearing aid (and earmould, in the case of a behind-the-ear style of aid) in the ear. Repeated attempts are often required before the client can insert and remove the aids satisfactorily. It is very often helpful if the client has a friend or relative present with them so that they can also see how the aid should look when in place in the ear (as well as providing support and additional memory for the client during the entire practical instruction). Where a client has difficulty in inserting or removing the aid, retraining is usually successful but earmould modifications may also be helpful, for example by:

- Cutting back the helix (top part) of the mould, which many clients find difficult to position correctly, see *Figure 5.7*
- Making a full shell earmould into a skeleton, see *Figure 5.7*; a skeleton has no central portion and can make inserting and removing the hearing aid easier
- Adding a removal handle.

Amplification

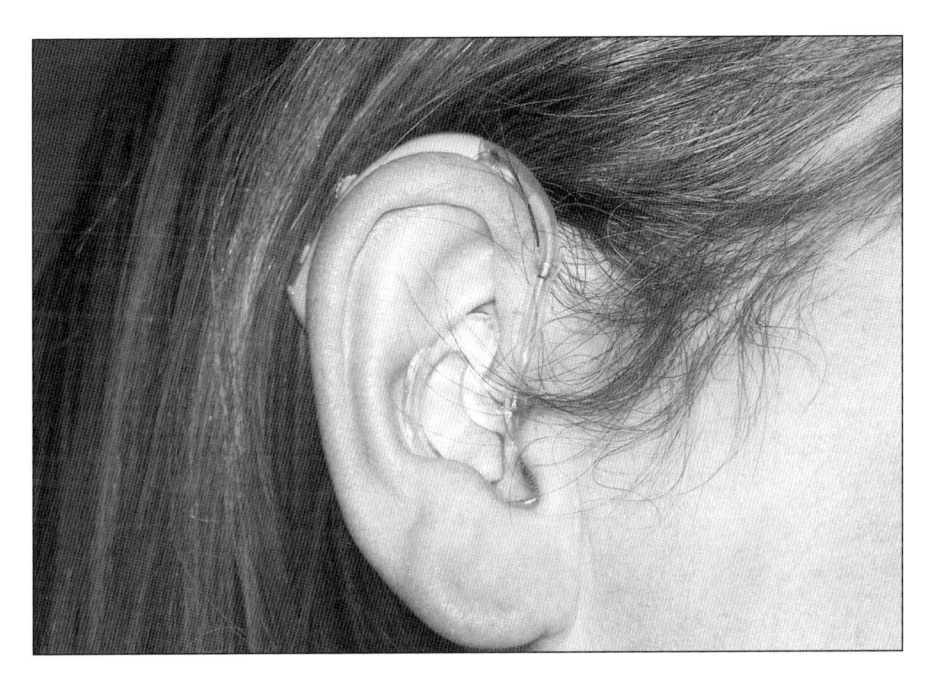

Figure 5.7 A skeleton earmould correctly inserted
(Reproduced with kind permission of Hannah Williams)

The client should understand acoustic feedback, when and why it happens and how to prevent it. Acoustic feedback is the high pitched whistle that occurs when sound from the outlet leaks back into the microphone and is re-amplified. A common cause of feedback is the reflection of the sound from a wax blockage in the ear, therefore the need to keep the ear clear of wax should be included in the discussion.

Simple cleaning and general care and maintenance of the hearing aids should be explained and demonstrated as appropriate:

- Handle the aids with clean, dry hands.
- Every day any wax should be removed from the sound

outlet and the vent, using wax removal tools, see *Figure 5.8*. A wax cleaning spray can be used if required.
- Wax traps should be replaced regularly, see *Figure 5.9*.

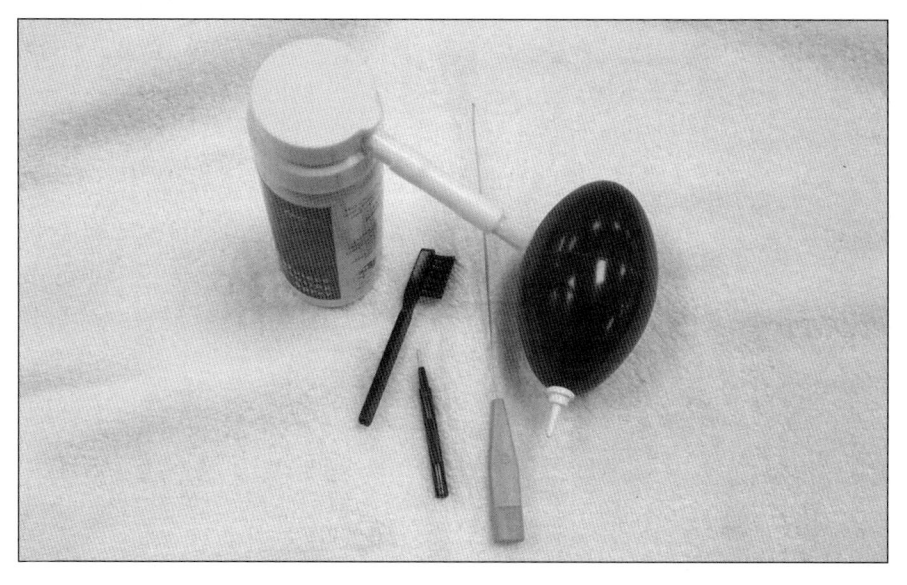

Figure 5.8 *Cleaning tools*

Amplification

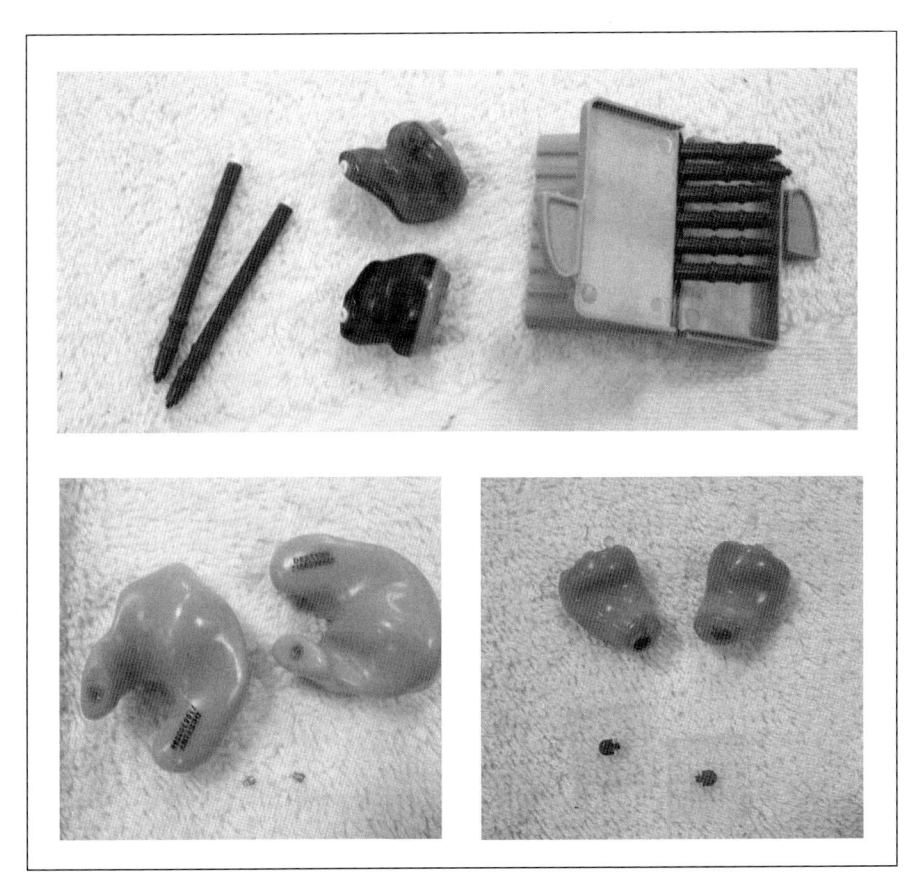

Figure 5.9 *Wax traps*

- The aid casing or 'housing' can be wiped using a clean damp cloth.
- If a behind-the-ear hearing aid is being worn, the earmould should be separated from the aid for washing in warm soapy water, once a week or more often if necessary. After washing, the earmould should be carefully dried and any water droplets removed, ideally using an air puffer to blow them out, as water in the tubing can cause intermittent sound to

reach the ear. The earmould should be reattached to the aid as shown in *Figure 5.10*.

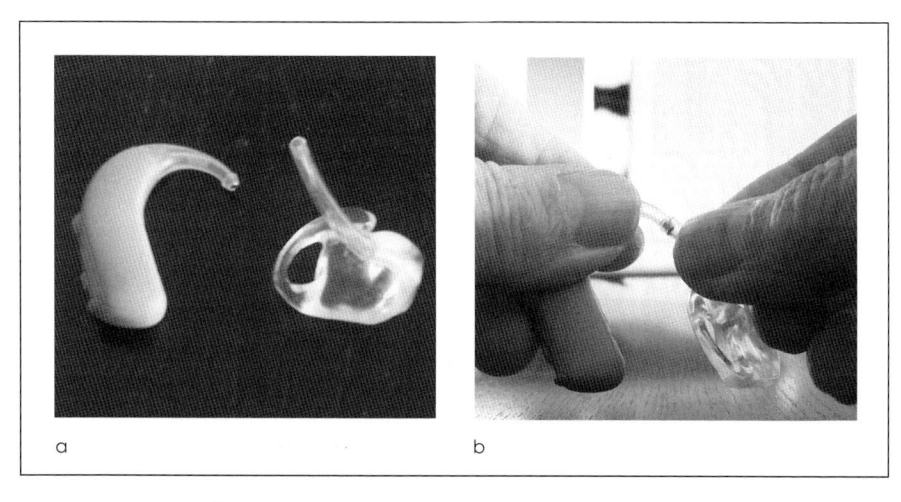

Figure 5.10 *Reattaching the earmould*
    (a) Lining the earmould up with the hearing aid
    (b) Attaching the tube to the earhook

- The aids should be turned off when they are not in use and, if they are not being used for a long period, the batteries should be removed.
- The aids should not be worn during the night when sleeping. The battery compartment should be left open. It is sensible to keep the aids in their protective case and to put them in the same safe place every night.
- The aids should be treated with care; they should not be dropped or exposed to extreme temperatures or humidity. They should not be worn in the bath or shower or when washing the hair or using hair spray.
- The aids and batteries should not be left where they may be picked up by small children or animals.

- Care should be taken with delicate moving parts such as the battery compartment. The battery compartment should not be forced to close; if it does not close, it is likely that the battery has not been inserted correctly.
- Dead batteries should always be removed and not left in the battery compartment.
- If the aid is of the behind-the-ear type, the tubing should be replaced, see *Figure 5.11*. This should be done before the tubing becomes hard or discoloured; if the earmould is made of silicone, the tubing should be replaced regularly, every few weeks, as the tubing tends to collapse within the earmould. If the aids are body worn, damaged leads or cords need replacing as they may provide intermittent sound.
- It is advisable to carry a spare battery when going out.

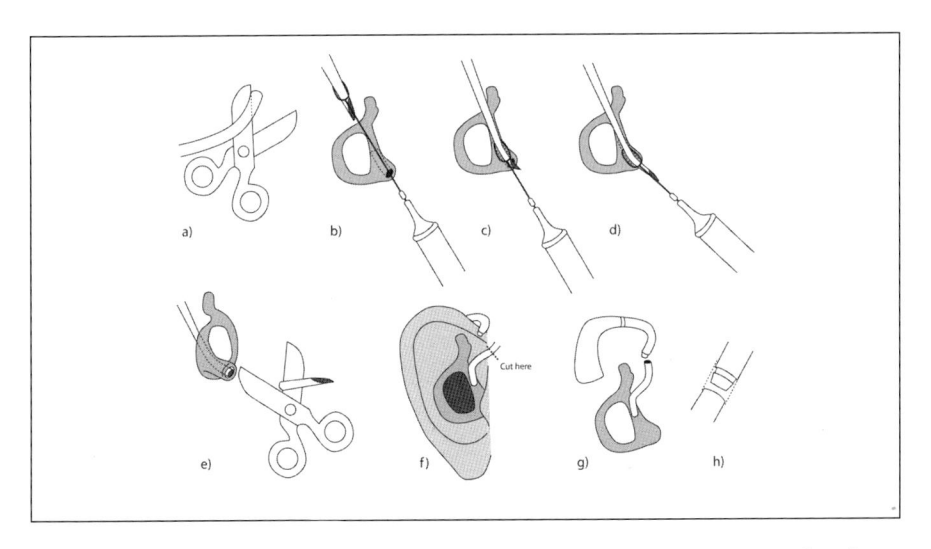

Figure 5.11 *Replacing tubing in an earmould (Reproduced with kind permission of Anglia Distance Learning Ltd)*

- An instruction booklet, see *Figure 5.12*, or a simple instruction leaflet should always be supplied as a great deal of information is given in a short period of time. Clients' questions should be answered and they should know how to obtain further assistance if and when required. A follow up appointment should also be arranged.

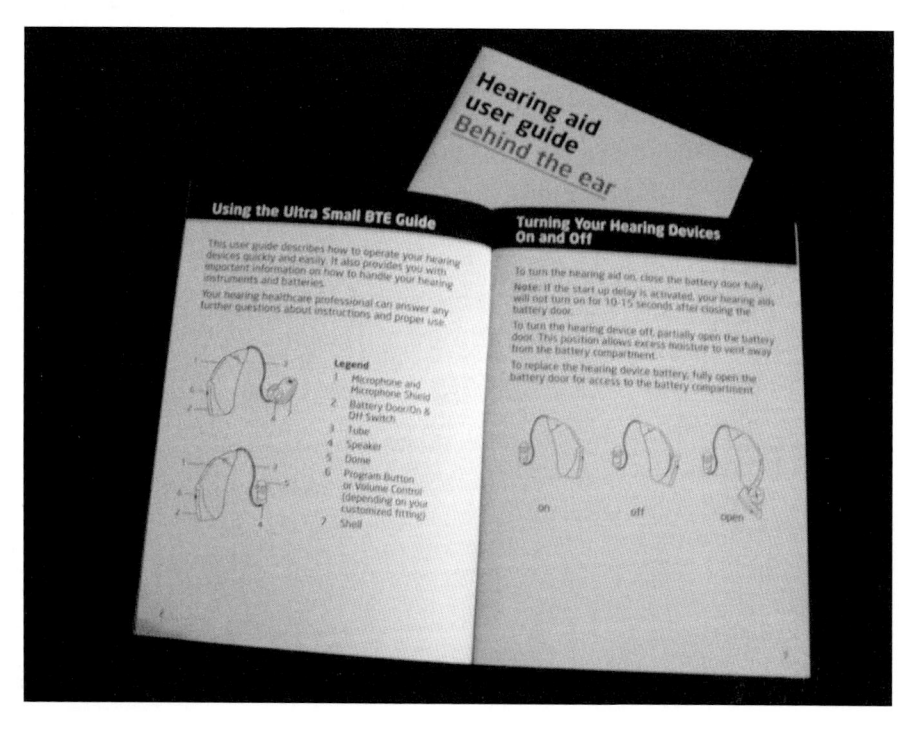

Figure 5.12 An instruction booklet

5.3.3 Becoming accustomed to wearing hearing aids

If the client has had a hearing loss for some time without aiding, it will take time to become accustomed to the sound of a noisy world again and the brain will need to re-learn to associate sounds with their meanings. New clients are unlikely to realise that hearing aids are not like spectacles, where the amount of adjustment to a new sensory perception is relatively minimal.

Readjustment is a gradual process although it will vary according to the character and age of the individual. Some people, especially younger adults, will feel able to use the aids all the time from the beginning but many people, particularly elderly clients, may find using the hearing aids very tiring at first. They will need to build up their use gradually. They should be encouraged to adopt a gradual, structured approach and, where appropriate, the time of use should be built up from short periods (e.g. an hour or two) in easy listening situations to more difficult situations for longer periods and eventually to wearing the aids all day, every day. The pace of rehabilitation should not be unnecessarily restricted for those who are able and keen, but anyone finding it difficult or tiring should be encouraged to use a structured approach, such as shown in *Figure 5.13*.

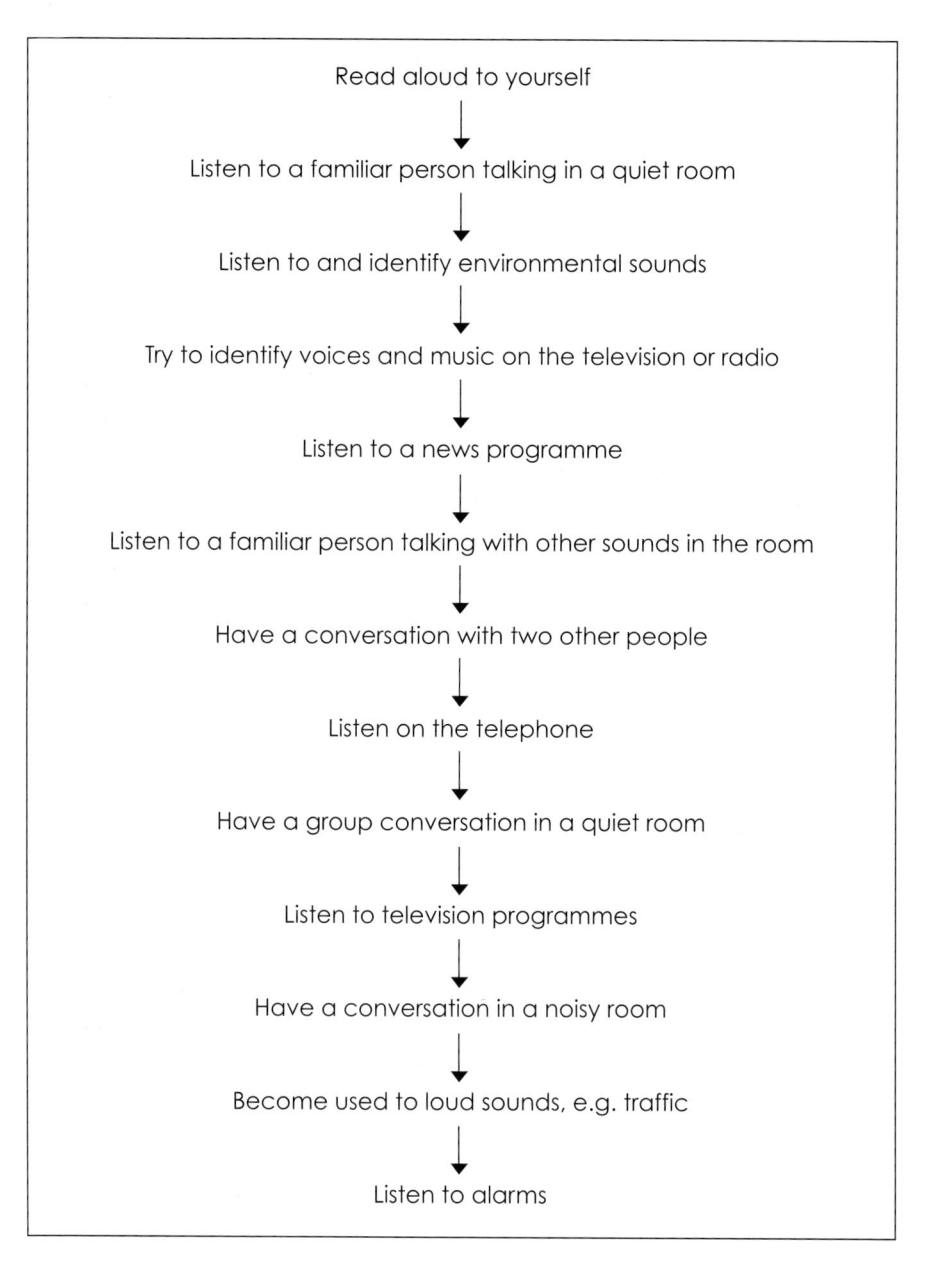

Read aloud to yourself
↓
Listen to a familiar person talking in a quiet room
↓
Listen to and identify environmental sounds
↓
Try to identify voices and music on the television or radio
↓
Listen to a news programme
↓
Listen to a familiar person talking with other sounds in the room
↓
Have a conversation with two other people
↓
Listen on the telephone
↓
Have a group conversation in a quiet room
↓
Listen to television programmes
↓
Have a conversation in a noisy room
↓
Become used to loud sounds, e.g. traffic
↓
Listen to alarms

Figure 5.13 An example of a planned programme of listening environments

An ability to differentiate sounds rapidly is needed to understand speech. It takes time, patience and effort to become familiarised with sound meaning patterns again after a prolonged period of hearing impairment. It is quite usual to need three months or more to benefit optimally from hearing aids. The client needs to understand that, even after such a period of rehabilitation, hearing will not return to 'normal'. Speech will be clearer but other sounds will also be amplified and some situations will always remain difficult, for example listening from another room or in reverberant conditions. In addition, the client should know that their own voice is likely to sound different and may seem as if it is echoing inside their head. It is very important that expectations of the hearing aids are realistic or disappointment, frustration and rejection of the hearing aids are likely to follow.

Many hearing aids provide a log of the amount of time the aids have been used and the settings at which they have been worn. This information can be very useful to the audiologist in recognising when problems exist, before it is too late to resolve them. There are three common usage patterns:

1. Hearing aid use is gradually built up over time. These clients usually become good full-time hearing aid users.
2. The hearing aids are used only briefly and then put aside. This may be due to some problem such as embarrassment, discomfort, handling difficulties, limited benefit or unrealistic expectations. If not tackled and overcome early on, the aids are likely to be permanently rejected.
3. Intermittent use. The client neither rejects the aid nor uses it full time. Usage is limited to those specific situations in which the client feels it is beneficial to them.

5.3.4 Hearing tactics

The aim of using hearing tactics is to minimise any environmental disadvantage that may create problems for the hearing impaired person. General advice may include:

1. Avoid or reduce background noise, e.g. by turning off the television or radio, by having a carpet instead of a hard floor or even by using a table cloth.
2. The room should be well lit and the light should fall on the speaker's face, not in the hearing impaired listener's eyes.
3. Be close to the speaker to minimise the loss of signal intensity over distance; about 1m is generally ideal for listening and speech reading.
4. Other people can help by addressing the hearing impaired person by name before they speak, facing them and speaking slowly and clearly rather than shouting. They should also be prepared to repeat or rephrase things that cause misunderstanding.

5.4 PRESCRIPTION TOLERANCE

In the early stages of getting used to a newly-prescribed hearing aid, whether it is an upgraded prescription or a new fitting to a first time user, there may be some intolerance to the required prescription. Sometimes it is necessary to 'tone down' the prescription in the early rehabilitation period and to build up to the full prescription gradually as the client adapts.

Chapter 6
A Psychosocial Framework

6.1 PSYCHOSOCIAL ISSUES

Deafness is the most common physical disability and can have a very significant psychological, social and economic impact on an individual's life. Typical problems are listed in *Table 6.1*.

Table 6.1 Typical problems encountered by a hearing impaired person

Problem	Description
A degree of paranoia	This develops as the hearing impaired person suspects that, because they cannot hear what is being said, people must be talking about them.
Conversational errors	Mistakes made in everyday conversation at work and at home. These can be embarrassing socially and may jeopardise employment or career advancement if the underlying problem is not recognised.
Becoming the butt of a joke	Fun may be made of the deaf person and even a non-malicious joke can be upsetting. Sometimes the deaf person may suspect they are the butt of a joke when it is not the case.

Table 6.1 Typical problems encountered by a hearing impaired person continued

Loss of desire to communicate verbally	Difficulties encountered in simply maintaining a conversation can make the sufferer an outcast.
Frustration	An inability to communicate may cause the deafened person to feel bitter, resentful and frustrated, which colleagues may interpret as being anti-social.
Employment restrictions	Depending upon the severity of the hearing loss and the individual's ability to overcome the handicap, certain employment may not be practical and a change of job may be necessary.

Deafness results in communication problems. Inappropriate responses to questions can be embarrassing and the individual may be, or at least feel, left out of discussions and family decisions. Communication with friends, family and colleagues and even simple daily activities, such as shopping, become more difficult. Work prospects, performance and satisfaction can all be affected. The everyday sounds that keep us in touch with our environment reduce or disappear. Not only conversation but also alerting sounds, such as the telephone or footsteps, and even background noises, such as general babble, traffic, the fridge or air conditioning are all part of our normal experience. Their removal can have a psychological effect bringing unreality, fear, loss of confidence and competence, isolation and loneliness.

People deal with deafness in different ways. Many deny hearing loss even to themselves and instead accuse others of mumbling or failing to speak clearly. Some people feel uncomfortable. They may fear rejection if they admit their deafness and they develop strategies to hide it. Some individuals become irritable, aggressive or dominating, especially when they cannot follow what is being said. Others simply withdraw from social situations.

Communication problems can cause strong emotional reactions. The deaf individual may feel isolation, frustration, anxiety, fear, embarrassment, stress and sensory deprivation. They may grieve for their lost hearing, for the loss of voices, music and environmental sounds, especially if the loss is sudden so there is no opportunity to adapt gradually. Depression, dependence and withdrawal are common reactions for those with acquired deafness. In fact, the emotional response to deafness can sometimes be more disabling than the deafness itself.

The communication problems also affect others and the way they think about and relate to the deaf person. Even close family members often tend to think that the deaf person is inattentive or 'hears when he wants to'. The impact on a partner is particularly significant. Their life also is affected by the communication difficulties. Roles change as the deaf person becomes more dependent and the significant other has to provide support. They may be unprepared for this and also find it difficult to cope. They may become overprotective or may resent having to relay conversations and feel they are missing out themselves by having to do this. They are likely to experience the same emotions, such as shock, anger and grief, as the hearing impaired individual, but they may also feel guilt. The guilt is usually unjustified and due to the demands, problems, limitations, expectations and responsibilities placed on them. Successful communication takes more effort on everyone's part and relationships can become very strained.

6.2 LOSS AND GRIEF

6.2.1 Stages of grief

Grief is a natural process which occurs for something that has been or would have been but is now lost. Grief can occur with any kind of loss. A deaf person may grieve for their loss of hearing or a parent may grieve for their unrealised dreams of a physically perfect child. Grief is a coping mechanism and is a way of facing the shock of an unwanted loss.

Grief is very real and needs to be worked through before acceptance and positive rehabilitation can be achieved. However, the effects of deafness are such that negative feelings may be reinforced every day and counselling may be needed to help the deaf person and their family. The audiologist needs to be aware of the feelings of loss which the client may experience and should help them through the grieving process with empathy and understanding.

The grieving process consists of a number of stages (Kubler-Ross, 2005) through which a person may pass in coming to terms with loss:

- *Denial* is a defence mechanism and a normal reaction to hearing loss. If deafness is rejected the painful reality does not have to be faced. Short-term denial acts as a self-protection and also allows the individual time to adjust to their new state. However protracted denial will prevent the individual from moving forward. Denial has to be resolved before coping behaviours can develop.
- *Anger* may follow as the second stage of the grieving process. The person asks 'Why me?' and feels the unjustness of it all. Anger is a normal defence mechanism but if protracted it can be very negative, delay

A Psychosocial Framework

rehabilitation and have a major impact on those close to the hearing impaired person.
- *Bargaining* is a mechanism that involves an attempt to find an improved outcome. It is a hopeful stage and may be realistic but more often is not. The individual often has unrealistic expectations and rehabilitation is unlikely to succeed until these have been replaced with realistic goals. If a client believes that hearing aids will restore perfect hearing for example, the likelihood is that the hearing aids will be rejected.
- *Depression* is a normal state but not a desirable one. When the individual realises they are unable to change the situation they are forced to accept the facts but feel helpless and depressed by them. If depression does not give way to more positive acceptance fairly rapidly, depression can spiral into a state where progress is almost impossible.
- *Acceptance* is the final stage of grief in which the individual accepts the reality of the situation and is ready to make positive decisions. Acceptance does not necessarily imply that the person is motivated but it is a stage at which the person can be motivated to do something about their hearing problems. They are ready to make goal-orientated decisions and to move on.

6.2.2 The change transition curve

The stages of grief can be shown as a change transition curve which can be used to describe the emotional stages that people are likely to experience with any life change. *Figure 6.1* shows the transition curve adapted for hearing loss. The curve shows the following stages:

1. *Denial of the loss of hearing:* This is the stage where other people are often blamed for any problems, for example "I can't understand you because you always mumble".
2. *Awareness:* This is an uncomfortable period, the hearing impaired person experiences frustration, anxiety and loss of control.
3. *Expectation:* This is the stage where someone offers a solution (usually hearing aids) but the client's expectations are often unrealistically high and they are very hopeful and optimistic.
4. *Acceptance of reality:* The client finds the hearing aids do not match up to their expectations and there are disappointments, for example perhaps their own voice sounds echoing or perhaps the aids are too visible or too noisy or do not give as much help as the client had envisaged. The client may fall into a pit of negative emotions: anger, aggression, withdrawal, depression. At this stage they may give up wearing the hearing aids, either through cancellation or putting them away in a drawer. The client needs help to focus on going forward but the problems seem too big and too much effort.
5. *Experimentation:* The audiologist needs to break the problems and objections down and create a rehabilitation plan with steps that the client can manage. It might, for example, consist of steps to build up wearing the aids from half an hour in quiet, to longer periods and then to gradually more difficult situations. The audiologist should also appreciate that clients often fail to explain the whole picture or tend to over-generalise, for example "I don't understand anyone" or "Everyone shouts at me". Questioning these assumptions should enable the audiologist to reach below the surface to clarify the client's objectives. For example, a client might say "It's

uncomfortable to wear" leading the audiologist to take a new impression, when the client's real complaint could be that they find it embarrassing to be seen wearing a hearing aid in public. A new earmould would not solve this problem but only make extra work. A more discreet aid might be an answer but improving the client's confidence and self esteem are likely to be as, or even more, important.

6. *Internalising*: This is where the client is now more comfortable with the hearing aids and using strategies and tactics to improve the communication environment. The client is beginning to identify with the transition and is generally positive.
7. *Integration*: The new behaviours are fully integrated into the person's life.

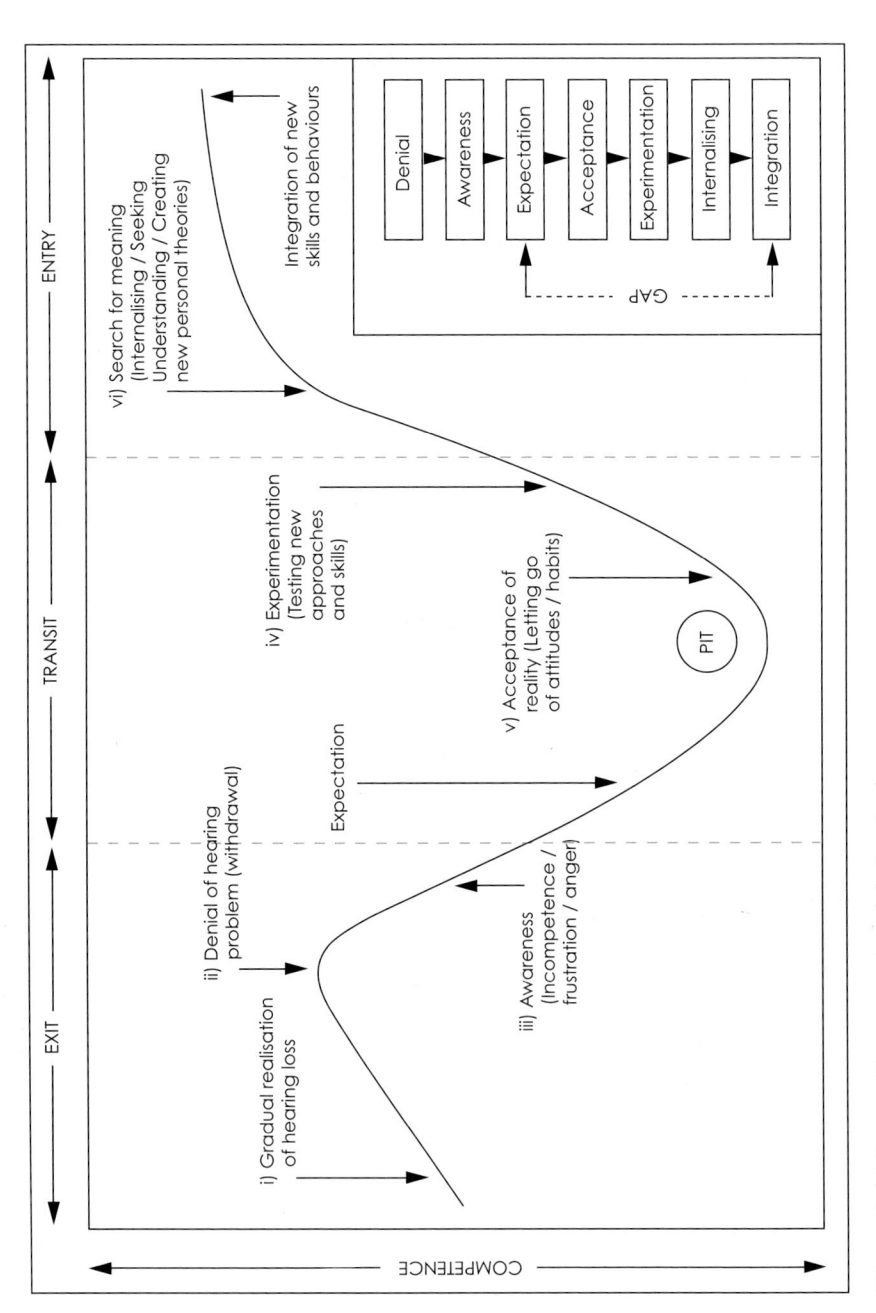

Figure 6.1 The transition curve adapted for hearing loss

The transition is made much more difficult when the client has unrealistic expectations, that is where a large gap exists between the expectations and the successful integration, see *Figure 6.2*. The rehabilitation process should aim to make the gap as small as possible by ensuring the client is made aware that hearing will not be restored to normal, of the sort of problems that may arise, and that it will take time to adjust to the hearing aids and to be able to make the most effective use of them. It is equally important that the client knows that they are not facing this alone as the audiologist will be there to help and support them along the way, for as long as their help is needed.

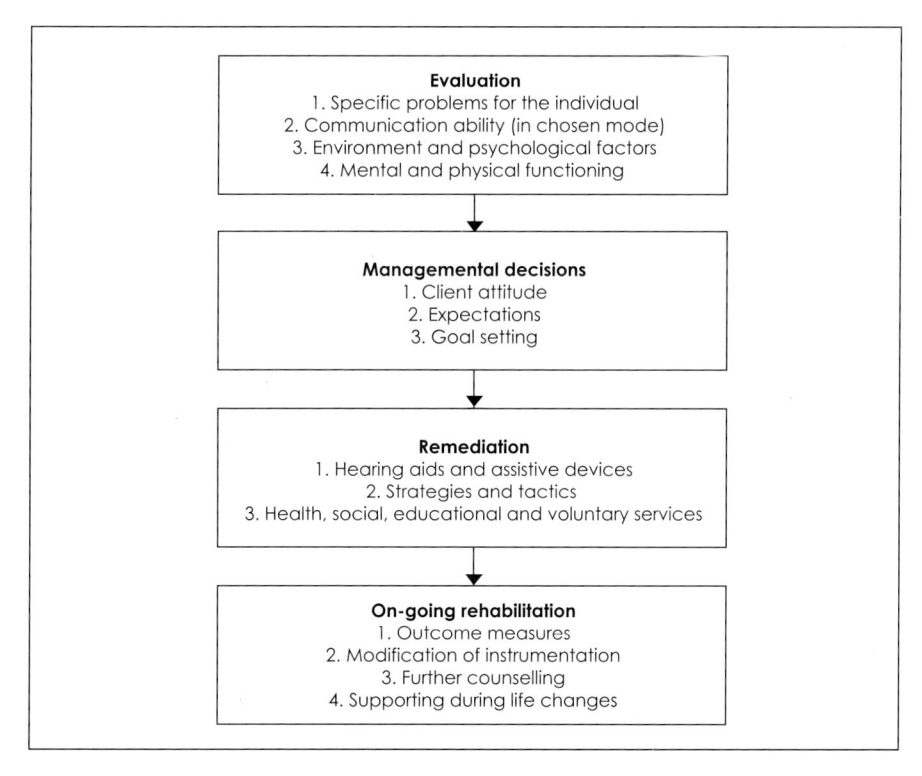

```
┌─────────────────────────────────────────────────┐
│              Evaluation                          │
│    1. Specific problems for the individual       │
│    2. Communication ability (in chosen mode)     │
│    3. Environment and psychological factors      │
│    4. Mental and physical functioning            │
└─────────────────────────────────────────────────┘
                        ↓
┌─────────────────────────────────────────────────┐
│          Managemental decisions                  │
│             1. Client attitude                   │
│             2. Expectations                      │
│             3. Goal setting                      │
└─────────────────────────────────────────────────┘
                        ↓
┌─────────────────────────────────────────────────┐
│              Remediation                         │
│    1. Hearing aids and assistive devices         │
│    2. Strategies and tactics                     │
│    3. Health, social, educational and voluntary services │
└─────────────────────────────────────────────────┘
                        ↓
┌─────────────────────────────────────────────────┐
│          On-going rehabilitation                 │
│          1. Outcome measures                     │
│       2. Modification of instrumentation         │
│          3. Further counselling                  │
│       4. Supporting during life changes          │
└─────────────────────────────────────────────────┘
```

Figure 6.2 *The rehabilitation process*

6.2.2.1 The transition curve

A Possible Patient Journey (Ida Institute, 2009) is a practical model that relates well to the change transition curve and which can be used by audiologists to chart each patient's unique experience. The model, see *Appendix*, explores previous, as well as potential future experiences to gain a fuller appreciation of an individual's rehabilitation 'journey' and increase the potential for positive outcomes.

Phases include:

- *Pre-Awareness* – The patient is experiencing communication problems but may be "managing" without acknowledging the hearing problem, they may also be bewildered or frustrated and their family and friends may begin to notice their hearing difficulties.

- *Awareness* – The patient realises that hearing loss is impacting on their social and work life. They may recognise the problem and begin to map the problems it causes and they may "self test" by raising TV volume or attempting to control other environmental sounds.

- *Movement* – The patient reaches a "tipping point" and is ready to consult a health care professional. They gather information about hearing loss from a variety of sources including their personal network, General Practitioner, the web and other media.

- *Diagnostics* – The patient actively seeks referrals to hearing care professionals and meets with them for interview and case history, hearing test and recommendations, leading to decision making.

- *Rehabilitation* – The patient takes action by seeking counselling, treatment and hearing aid fitting and/or considers other assistive devices. In this context, the patient develops a communication strategy that leads to acceptance or rejection of the recommendations of the hearing care professional.

- *Post-Clinical* – The patient undergoes a process of adaptation and change. They observe the social impact and continue to self-evaluate the success or failure of the treatment outcome. Either the problem is resolved or the patient now becomes aware of new problems.

6.2.3 Hierarchy of need

A person may not be able to move on with the rehabilitation programme if they have more basic needs. Maslow (1968) suggested a hierarchy of five levels of need, which is depicted as a pyramid in *Figure 6.3*. A person can only concentrate on higher needs if the more pressing (lower) needs have been satisfied. Physiological needs are those of life and survival. Safety needs are those which provide structure and security, for example home, work, etc. The next level is that of love and belonging. If a client is facing problems at any of these levels (particularly the first two) it may not be an appropriate time to consider hearing aids.

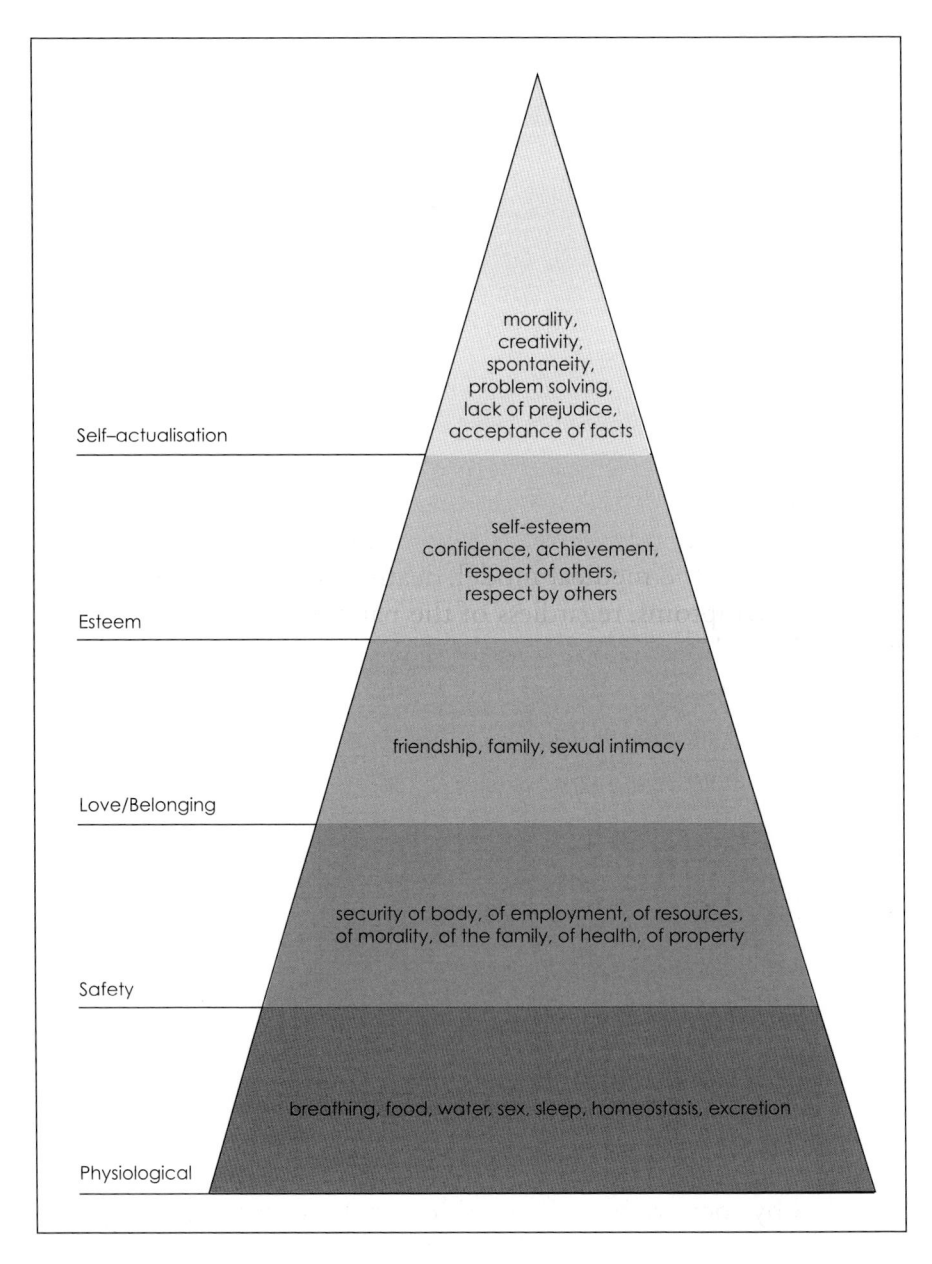

Figure 6.3 *Maslow's hierarchy of need*

6.3 DISABILITY AND HANDICAP

Despite disability laws, our society still tends to devalue disabled people and disabled lifestyles. Four models of disability are outlined below: medical, social, bio-psychosocial and cultural.

(1) The medical model

The medical model assumes that people with disabilities are 'sick' and need to be cured by doctors. All responsibility for treatment lies with medical professionals, who will diagnose and treat the disability. Medical professionals become the decision makers who give instruction on how to resolve the problem, with the individual becoming a passive recipient of treatment and charity. In the medical model, deafness is considered as a cluster of symptoms, regardless of the patient's lifestyle, personality, education and other psychological and social factors.

Audiometric evaluation and hearing aid fitting is still widely viewed as a medical field. The client is taught how to cope with the 'disease' and is responsible only for co-operating. Client counselling is often seen as less important than diagnosis although in reality it could be that technological advances are, at least sometimes, less important to success than rehabilitative counselling (Hawkins, 1990).

(2) The social model of disability

In the 1960s and 70s, there was a movement away from the 'medical model' towards human rights and the inclusion of disabled people. A distinction began to be made between impairment (e.g. hearing loss) and disability (the restrictions imposed by society, through prejudice, lack of understanding, insufficient resources, etc.). The World Health Organisation

(WHO) provided a framework for this in its International Classification of Impairments, Disabilities and Handicaps (1980). The term 'social model of disability' was introduced in the early 1980s (Oliver, 1983).

The social (or disability) model views disability as constructed by society. It is society's attitudes and prejudices, barriers and exclusions (such as restricted access to education and work environments and to social support services) that create the disability, rather than the actual impairment. Attempts to 'cure' or improve the individual (especially against their wishes) imply that the person is of less value. This is therefore considered to show prejudice and discrimination. The social model seeks to overcome the social barriers and promotes disability rights, equality, independence and inclusion. Removal of the barriers empowers people with disabilities to make their own decisions, to participate in and contribute to society, and to be seen as equal.

'Being deaf is not about being disabled, or medically incomplete – it's about being part of a linguistic minority. We're proud, not of the medical aspect of deafness, but of the language we use and the community we live in.' (Garfield, 2006).

Many of the deaf signing population consider themselves as a separate community with its own language. They argue that sign language should be valued in the same way as the spoken language of an ethnic group. Many view the cochlear implantation of deaf children as undesirable because these children will probably not become part of the 'Deaf community'. The social model seeks to accommodate the different needs and goals.

The social model is reflected in our current disability laws, which require the removal of barriers and the promotion of equality. The World Health Organisation has replaced its earlier classification with the International Classification of Functioning, Disability and Health (2001) which views disability as a universal human experience and shifts the focus from cause to impact.

(3) The bio-psychosocial model

The bio-psychosocial model was introduced by Engel (1977) to link biological, psychological and social factors (*Figure 6.4*) which all impact upon recovery. He believed that the 'medical model must also take into account the patient, the social context in which he lives' and society's healthcare system. The bio-psychosocial model views disability as a part of normal life that should be integrated into everyday activities rather than having to be 'overcome'.

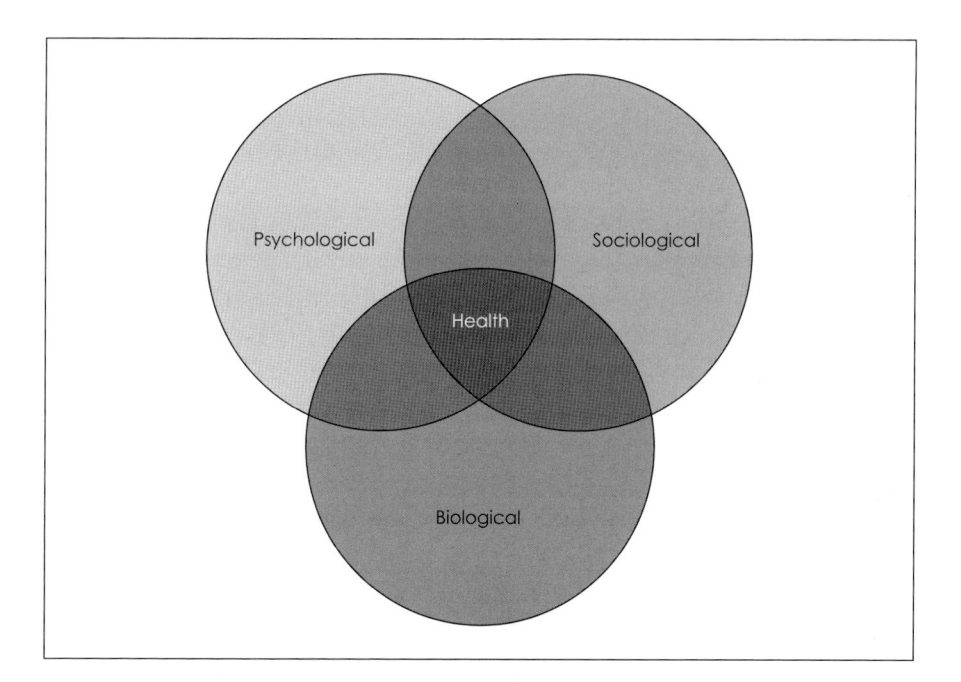

Figure 6.4 Engel's bio-psychosocial model

(4) The cultural model

The cultural model embraces disability rather than seeking to 'overcome' it. Within the cultural model, disability is a state of being and the emphasis is on issues of human and civil rights.

The Deaf community have developed their own culture and do not regard themselves as disabled. Instead they see themselves as a linguistic minority (similar to an ethnic minority) whose first language is signed. Deaf culture has its own language and social and cultural norms, which are different from those of the hearing community. The Deaf are proud of their language and their community. Deafness is not seen as a disability, deficiency or handicap but as a culture (Lane, 1992, 1996; Parasnis, 1996) with its own theatre, art and literature. The term 'Deaf' (with a capital D) is a term of cultural identity and does not indicate any specific degree of deafness. Most members of the Deaf community are pre-lingually deaf but membership also extends to include others such as many children of deaf parents and some sign language interpreters.

6.4 THEORY AND APPLICATION OF REHABILITATIVE COUNSELLING

6.4.1 Steps in managing rehabilitative change

Change can be managed in a number of stages (Judson, 1991; Di Clemente et al, 1991; Morera et al, 1998; Prochaska and Di Clemente, 1983) that can basically be reduced to three (see *Figure 6.1*):

1. *Exit*: involves overcoming defence mechanisms and departing from the existing state. This stage will involve analysing, planning and communicating the change.

2. *Transit*: is typically a period of confusion as old ways are challenged. This stage will involve gaining acceptance of the change.
3. *Entry*: is where a new equilibrium is achieved. This stage involves changing to, and consolidating, the desired state.

Sanders (1993) suggests the following steps will be involved in managing rehabilitative change:

1. Provision of information and emotional support
2. Review and interpretation of test results
3. Identification of the current situation and needs
4. Obtaining supplementary information
5. Determining goals
6. Identifying resources
7. Developing a management plan
8. Monitoring the effectiveness of the programme.

In counselling clients through the basic steps and stages, the audiologist should be aware of counselling theory and techniques. The many approaches to counselling can be grouped under psychoanalytic, cognitive-behavioural or experiential theories.

6.4.2 Approaches based on psychoanalytic theory

Freudian theory was based on the existence of the id, ego and super-ego. The id is present at birth and is concerned with achieving instant gratification. The ego is the reality agent that mediates between the needs of the id for instant gratification and the external forces of reality. The super-ego is an internal system of values or morals that develops out of an awareness that some behaviours receive approval and others do not.

Psychoanalytic theory considers that maladjusted behaviour stems from excessive anxiety. The ego seeks to maintain a balance between the id and the super-ego so that the individual is not stressed and can function productively. The ego can use problem-solving strategies consciously to maintain the balance, or unconscious defence mechanisms to deny reality. Freudian defence mechanisms include, for example, displacement (transfer of emotions to a safe target) or repression (denying the existence of an anxiety-causing impulse).

Freudian theory has been discredited but modifications of it by others, such as Jung and Adler, led to the development of various approaches to psychoanalysis, psychotherapy and counselling. Psychoanalysis consists of taking an extended (often over several months) history and gaining insight into the client's problems by encouraging them to project their feelings onto the psychoanalyst. Psychotherapy is again a long-term strategy and it attempts to move the client's unconscious defence mechanisms into conscious awareness, where they can be confronted, understood and replaced with more positive strategies. Counselling addresses only certain ego mechanisms rather than the whole personality and is therefore a shorter process. It does not investigate unconscious memories of the past, as would psychoanalysis and psychotherapy, but seeks to strengthen the weakened ego and replace undesirable behaviours with adaptive, goal-orientated ones.

6.4.3 Approaches based on cognitive-behavioural theory

Behaviourists, such as Thorndike, Watson, Skinner and Eysenck, believed that psychology should be scientific, objective and observable. The behaviourist view of problem solving is a process of trial and error and was based on animal experiments. Through his experiments Thorndike established three 'laws of learning':

1. *The law of effect* states that, once a connection has been made between a behaviour and an outcome, a reward will strengthen that behaviour and a punishment will weaken it; rewards being more important than punishments.
2. *The law of readiness* states that the connection will only be satisfying for the animal if they are ready for it, in which case they will try to maintain it. If they are not ready, they will attempt to eliminate it.
3. *The law of exercise* states that connections are strengthened through practice and weakened through disuse. Practice followed by rewards are of most importance.

According to behaviourists, behaviour can be explained through reference to observable stimuli, with no emphasis placed on the role of meaning or understanding.

Behaviour modification refers to a number of techniques based on behaviourist theory and uses the principles of conditioning. Conditioning involves the association of a response with a stimulus; reinforcement and punishment (operant conditioning) can be used to change behaviour. Rewarding appropriate behaviour is central to behaviour modification techniques. Behaviour that is reinforced is more likely to occur again, whilst behaviour that is punished may weaken. Conditioning methods can be used in behavioural counselling; this is a directive approach in which the professional works with the client to guide them gradually towards the desired goals.

Cognitive psychology is concerned with internal mental processes, such as memory, and language, and how people use these mental processes to solve problems. Cognitive theory is based on the premise that how we think determines how we feel. Self-defeating thoughts and behaviours, based on irrational beliefs, can prevent or impede positive development in the counselling process. Cognitive therapy therefore questions the assumptions a client has made and explores the reasons for them. It can then help the client to reach a realistic view. Small but significant linguistic changes, such as using 'I want to' (or 'I don't want to') instead of 'I should', or 'and' instead of 'but', and other techniques, such as role play, can show the client that their fears are irrational, introduce new more rational and adaptive patterns of thinking and, in addition, place the responsibility for actions and choices on the client.

6.4.4 Approaches based on experiential theory

Experiential theory suggests that there is more to problem solving than just trial and error. Perception is based on the entire situation and problem solving examines the relationship between the individual components and the whole problem.

Prior knowledge and novel solutions are both utilised in finding solutions.
People often struggle to find solutions to their problems because they have become biased by their experiences and therefore favour a problem-solving technique based on prior knowledge, or they may simply fail to see the possibility of a novel solution. There are various experiential approaches, all of which are based on restructuring the problems in order to find a solution.
Client-centred (or person-centred) counselling (Rogers, 1951) rests on the premise that individuals are inherently rational and goal-directed and that they have the basic capacity to control their own destiny. Everyone has an internal frame of reference formed from their perception of the environment. All behaviour is purposeful and in response to perceived reality, defensive behaviours are developed against threats to the self. Anything which is inconsistent with the self's values may be falsified, distorted or denied. If the defensive behaviours are insufficient to

A Psychosocial Framework

maintain the equilibrium, the individual will develop anxiety and stress. In client-centred counselling, the experiences that have led to feelings of anxiety and stress must be identified and challenged. New positive behaviours must be learned and used to replace the old negative behaviours. Anyone can change if the right atmosphere of trust and respect is created and it is the role of the professional to create an environment of empathy and unconditional positive regard, in which behavioural change can occur.

The counsellor should show interest and try to identify with the client's experiences. They should not judge the client but should accept the person without conditions and they should foster trust through expression of their own perceptions, both negative and positive. The counsellor may also provide general goals but rehabilitation will be most successful if the specific goals and methods used are determined by the individual, i.e. the client should be enabled to find their own solutions.

Existential psychology or therapy views the client as a unique individual who is central to their own world of experiences. The relationship between the therapist and the client is more important than the techniques used, although the therapist may use more direct and confrontational methods than in client-centred counselling. In existential therapy, the client is helped to experience their own uniqueness in terms of both freedom and responsibility. The client is free to choose and to control their life – although with freedom comes responsibility.

The therapist also helps the client to see the difference between normal and neurotic forms of guilt and anxiety. Normal anxiety is proportionate to its cause and normal guilt occurs when the client violates society's rules. Neurotic anxiety is not a proportionate emotion and neurotic guilt occurs when someone perceives they are responsible for something which is outside their control. Existential therapy helps the client to distinguish between normal and neurotic emotions and to change from a neurotic state to a normal one.

The Gestalt approach shares many of the features of client-centred and existential therapies. It differs in that it is based on the theory that stimuli will always be organised into a pattern and perceived as a whole. The thoughts, perceptions and emotions can only be understood by considering them in the context of a whole person. The approach uses dialogue to explore the client's experiences.

There are various techniques that may be used to develop self-awareness, independence and self-regulation, for example personalising the dialogue by using personal pronouns, converting questions to statements, verbalising acceptance of responsibility for opinions, role play and role reversal.

6.4.5 The audiologist's approach to counselling

The audiologist's approach to counselling may be based on one particular theory, alternatively aspects of the various theories can be blended into a personal counselling framework. Whatever approach is adopted, it needs to be flexible so that it can be adjusted to suit the individual client. The most widely used approach to rehabilitation is based on client-centred problem solving. The audiologist develops a supportive relationship with the client in which they can find out about the client's lifestyle, beliefs and behaviours. The client is fully involved in all decision-making and the audiologist helps them to work through their social and emotional barriers so that they can come to recognise, understand and accept their hearing loss and to develop the knowledge, skills and confidence to address their difficulties.

Chapter 7
Communication and Auditory Training

7.1 CONVERSATIONAL ABILITY

Auditory training usually includes perceptual training, lip-reading and listening skills, which, together with coping skills, will contribute to success in using hearing aids and assistive devices.

Conversation is shared communication. Everyone uses rules when conversing to ensure that the topic is shared, that one person does not do all the talking and that the information communicated is relevant and sufficient but without being too verbose. Turn-taking is an important part of conversational skill and the most fluent exchanges tend to be those that involve taking relatively equal turns. Communication rules are known subconsciously and even babbling babies can be heard to take turns with their mothers. Unfortunately hearing impairment can disrupt the use of conversational rules.

In an attempt to cope with their communication difficulties, many hearing impaired individuals develop maladaptive strategies, such as pretending to understand, ignoring what has been said or talking too much (generally to avoid having to listen). There are a number of reasons why people act in these ways including not wanting to let others know they have a hearing loss, not wanting to disrupt the conversation, not having the repair strategies or the energy to use them or not knowing the conversation partner well enough to feel able to assert their needs.

Erber (1996) suggests that hearing impaired people often display the following:

- Disrupted turn-taking
- Modified speaking style
- Inappropriate shift of topic
- Superficial content
- Frequent clarification.

Conversational ability depends very much on the conversational setting, the situation, the topic and the partner. Communication strategies are actions taken to ease communication or correct problems that have occurred. The client can then be trained to modify the listening and speaking behaviours of others. An assertive communication style is generally helpful in this.

7.2 CONVERSATIONAL STYLE

Conversational style may be passive, assertive or aggressive (Kaplan et al, 1985). Someone using a *passive style* tends to avoid social interaction whenever possible and when engaged in conversation will often pretend to understand. An *assertive style* is one in which responsibility is taken for managing communication problems, using a considerate manner. An *aggressive style* involves hostile and sometimes dominating behaviour which is not pleasant in a conversation partner!

There is no communication style that is always right and the style will vary according to the situation. Most people are probably unaware of their communication style but it is important for hearing impaired people to understand the different styles and to appreciate that an assertive style tends to be most beneficial when they need to achieve conversational modifications to assist their understanding.

7.3 COMMUNICATION STRATEGIES

7.3.1 Communication training

Communication training should work on the factors that affect communication, which are:

1. The speaker,
2. The environment,
3. The listener, and
4. The message.

The client should be fully involved and activities such as brainstorming and directed discussion are preferable to lecturing or using printed materials, although printed materials and other media may be used to support training sessions.

Training might start, for example, by identifying situations where problems arise in the client's everyday life and assessing how effectively they use communication strategies in these settings. A list may be created of instructional strategies that the client feels their conversational partners could use. Some of these (perhaps four or five) can be selected as being those that the client (not the audiologist!) considers would be most important to their understanding. The audiologist can guide the client but they must have ownership of decisions if the strategies are to be put it into practice.

Such strategies might include acknowledging the hearing loss and asking the speaker to face them, to get their attention before speaking and to speak clearly and slightly slower than usual but not to shout or, in a group situation, requesting that individual members speak one at a time.

The strategies can be put into practice in a structured setting, for example through role play with the audiologist or the family member or even videoed scenarios, followed by evaluation and suggestions for improvement. With increased self-confidence, the client can then try the strategies in real life and report back on their success and failure, which can then be discussed.

7.3.2 Communication repair

It has been found (Collins & Blood (1990) and Blood & Blood (1999)) that, in general, people who acknowledge their disability are viewed as more likeable, sincere and reliable and better conversational partners than those with disabilities who provide no such acknowledgement. It is therefore important for the audiologist to guide and support the client so that they feel able to acknowledge their problems in this way.

When communication breaks down, further strategies are needed to repair the conversation. The starting point could again be noting strategies already used by the client (this could be based on a role play noisy situation), leading on to discussion of these and introduction and practice of more effective strategies.

Constant interruption of a speaker is irritating and disruptive so it is important for the client to develop the most effective strategies; these tend to be direct requests for confirmation or rephrasing. Specific strategies could include asking for:

- Indication of the topic
- Confirmation
- Repetition
- Simplification
- Rephrasing
- Elaboration
- An alternative form, such as in writing.

Non-specific repair strategies (e.g. asking for repetition by saying 'Pardon?' or 'What?') can appear in the short-term to be less disruptive than asking for rephrasing. However, the latter is generally much more likely to result in understanding and therefore less likely to interrupt the flow of conversation. The client may benefit from examples of the kind of request or comment they could make, such as:

- Can you wait a minute for me to turn the television off? I can hear better with less noise.
- Could you slow down a bit? I find it hard to keep up with you.
- Did you say that …?
- I'll just repeat that back to you to make sure I heard you correctly.

Providing feedback to the conversation partner is also important, so that they know when what they are doing is helping the situation. Of course different strategies will be used in different situations. The choice will depend on how useful certain strategies have been found in the past, how much of the message was not understood and also on the perceived willingness of the conversation partner to assist.

7.3.3 Training the communication partner

The client may frequently need to rely on understanding and empathy from their communication partner. The partner's needs are therefore also very important and should not be forgotten. A partner too is affected by communication breakdowns and misunderstandings; they also can be isolated and lonely. The role of empathy and support is a tiring one and both partners may well become upset or angry. Counselling and training of the partner jointly with the client is usually helpful as the partner also requires support, whilst needing to understand how difficult and tiring speech reading is, and how they can help the communication process. Partners also can learn to:

- Avoid background noise
- Ensure their face can be clearly seen
- Speak naturally but slowly and clearly
- Simplify and keep to the point
- Use words that are easy to lipread
- Check understanding and rephrase when necessary.

7.3.4 Group training

Group training and self-help groups can provide an opportunity for the client to realise that they are not alone. In group sessions, clients may also watch others and identify and evaluate which repair strategies appear to be most effective or most ineffective. Speech reading skills and communication strategies can be practised in a safe and supportive environment. Information given individually can be repeated in the group and such repetition, together with listening to the comments and questions of others, can help the client towards increased understanding and acceptance. Involving the client's partner or other close family member or friend in the group sessions will help them to understand the problems and how they also can help in overcoming them.

The room to be used for training should be prepared before the session, for example ensuring that the furniture is arranged to facilitate easier communication, that the lighting is good and that glare is removed. It should be comfortable and warm but not too hot. If a loop system (see assistive devices, Chapter 11) is being used this, together with any other audiovisual equipment, should be set up and checked to make sure it is working, before the start of the meeting. Seating is often arranged either as a semicircle or, if tables are also being used, as a square or rectangle. To sit at tables may make new members of the group feel more secure and will give them somewhere to rest their worksheets and any drinks.

Group training should be planned and will usually be most successful if it involves techniques (such as brainstorming, directed discussion and role play) that fully involve the participants and are relevant to their real-life experiences. Each session should be organised to meet specified aims and objectives, see *Table 7.1*. Aims are overarching whereas objectives are bite-sized and can be written in the form 'By the end of the session, participants will be able to....'

Table 7.1 Examples of aims and objectives

Aims	Objectives
To manage stressful situations	• To list five stressful situations • To identify the symptoms of stress • To carry out a relaxation technique
To become more assertive	• To understand the difference between being assertive and being aggressive • To maintain appropriate eye contact throughout a conversation • To take responsibility for communication needs • To explain their hearing problem to others

The programme will normally be similar to an individual programme in that it will involve problem identification, exploration and resolution, see *Table 7.2*. The length of the training sessions and of the period over which sessions are held will vary according to the needs of the group but, for example, sessions might be one to two hours and held weekly for four to six weeks with perhaps a follow up meeting after three or four months.

Table 7.2 Items that will often be involved in the programme

1. Problem identification	2. Problem exploration	3. Problem resolution
Poor intelligibility	The audiogram	Speech reading practice
Everyday listening situations	Talking about deafness	Communication strategies
Difficult listening situations	Listing difficult situations	Assertiveness Assistive listening device
Emotional awareness	The effects of stress	Relaxation

Key factors covered in each meeting should be summarised towards the end of that meeting and the group should be praised for their involvement. Each session will usually involve some homework when the strategies that have been learned can be practised. Meetings should be evaluated and future sessions should be planned or revised according to the responses obtained. After the final weekly session, each participant should go away with a list of things they will try to achieve, for example:

I will tell other people that I have a hearing problem
I will wear my hearing aids all day
I will look at people when they are speaking to me
I will ask people to slow down or rephrase when I need them to
I will find out about a loop system for my lounge

At the follow-up meeting the success of the group in achieving their individual objectives can be discussed, together with any need for further help.

7.4 AUDITORY TRAINING

7.4.1 Auditory training programmes

Hearing is not the same as listening. Listening involves concentration in order to extract meaning from what is heard. Hearing aids do not restore normal function and do not, by themselves, make a person a good listener or communicator. An auditory training programme concentrates on listening skills with the aim of training the client to make full use of whatever sound cues are still available through their residual (remaining) hearing with appropriate amplification. Formal individual auditory training programmes tend to be used mainly with people who are severely and profoundly deaf, although some auditory training, to develop skill in perception, identification, discrimination and understanding, can be beneficial with any degree of hearing loss. *Figure 7.1* indicates possible stages of an auditory training programme. The less severe the hearing loss, the higher up the pyramid the individual will normally start.

Older adults will take longer to learn than younger adults (Bienfield, 1990) and may be less flexible in their learning style. They may need to concentrate on one task at a time but with increased patience, effort and practice can often learn as much as younger adults (Davis, 1990).

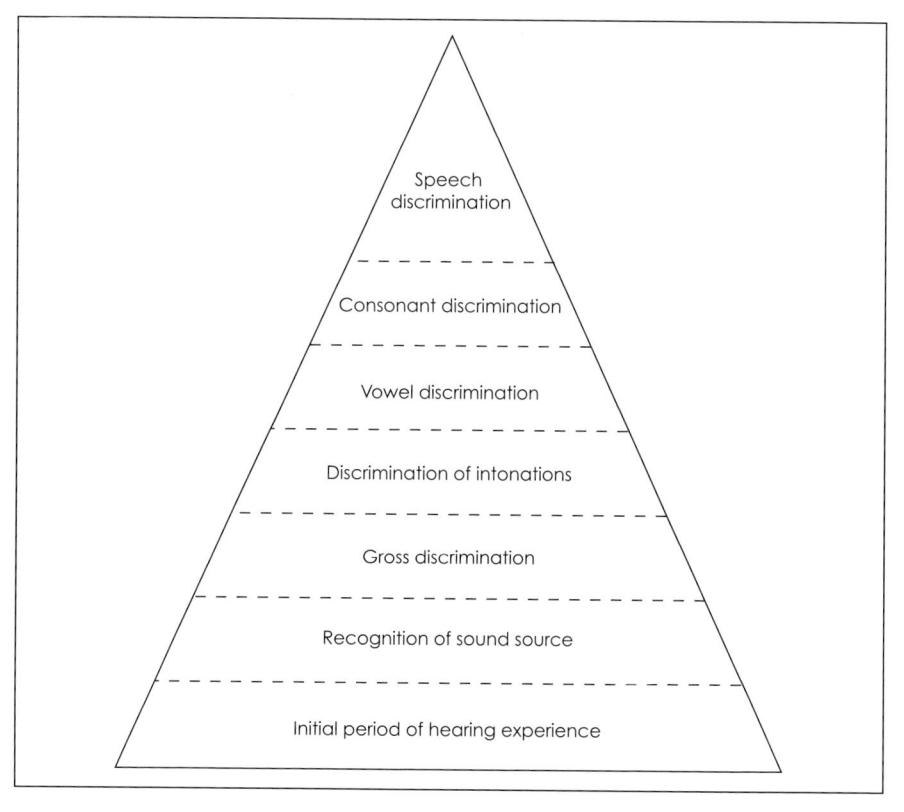

```
              Speech
              discrimination

           Consonant discrimination

          Vowel discrimination

       Discrimination of intonations

         Gross discrimination

       Recognition of sound source

     Initial period of hearing experience
```

Figure 7.1 An auditory training pyramid

Hearing impairment interferes with auditory feedback (hearing oneself speak) and can result in distorted speech patterns, especially of consonants, and an inappropriate voice level (usually too loud). An auditory training programme will usually include a series of exercises planned to help develop or maintain auditory memory, speech recognition and discrimination and will also normally include listening, decision making and responding. Tasks will become increasingly difficult as the participant progresses through the programme and should support the person in mastering the next step. Memory activities might include practice in concentrating and remembering names, through association for example. Speech recognition activities can be practised as exercises, games or in role play and might, for instance involve:

- Awareness of the presence and absence of sound
- Identification of environmental sounds
- Training in vowel recognition
- Practice related to rhythm and intonation
- Identification of phonemes
- Discrimination of words
- Understanding speech discourse
- Exercises in using context
- Practise with different accents.

The auditory training programme will usually include formal exercises to improve awareness and identification of sounds, discrimination of phonemes (speech sounds) and comprehension of sentences and running speech. Concentration and observation are very important and exercises should be included to develop attention to visual and spoken information, including rhythm, intonation and accent. Auditory memory can be improved with practice and memory exercises can help.

Speech Tracking, also called Continuous Discourse Tracking, may be used for training and evaluating ongoing speech. It involves someone reading a prepared text, a phrase at a time, for a set period, usually five or ten minutes. The listener has to repeat each phrase. If they are unable to do so, the speaker may repeat it or may apply other strategies such as rephrasing, but the next phrase will be introduced only when the listener has repeated the original segment exactly, word for word. At the end of the time period, the number of words repeated correctly is divided by the time, to give a score or tracking rate in words per minute (wpm). Normal tracking rates for the hearing population are around 100 wpm (De Filippo, 1988). Continuous Discourse Tracking can be a useful training and evaluation technique and has been used in this way with both adults (Plant, 1996) and children (Tye-Murray, 1998). The technique can be used in a modified version, for example Plant (1996) modified the procedure by using simple stories broken into parts of 200 words each. These are presented in small segments of 4 to 12 words at a time. The listener has to repeat as many words as possible but is allowed to use repair strategies in the case of difficulty. The score is the number of words correctly identified expressed as a percentage.

Auditory training sometimes includes special techniques, for example copying the movements of the articulators (lips, teeth, tongue, etc.) using touch and vision to produce correct speech sounds, or matching speech patterns to those displayed on a laryngograph screen, or computer-based training methods. Computer-based programmes can provide self-paced perceptual training in an environment chosen by the client.

7.4.2 Examples of computer-based auditory training programmes

i) Listening and Communication Enhancement (LACE) (Sweetow and Henderson-Sabes, 2004).

LACE is designed for use with any clients who report problems in understanding speech in difficult listening situations (with or without hearing loss). The training period is intended to last four weeks and it can therefore be completed within a client's hearing aid trial period. The programme aims to engage the client in the hearing aid fitting process, develop listening

Communication and Auditory Training

strategies, build confidence and address the cognitive changes associated with the ageing process.

There are twenty 30 minute sessions of graded exercises in:

1. *Understanding degraded speech*: Sentences are presented in background babble, with a competing speaker or as rapid (time compressed) speech. The client has to repeat the sentence (aloud or silently). The sentence is then presented visually and the client is asked if they understood it. If the response is affirmative the next sentence will be more difficult, and vice versa.

2. *Cognitive tasks*: Sentences are presented with a word masked by a random environmental sound, such as a car horn. The client has to select a word to replace it, from a short list. A short-term memory exercise is also introduced in which the client is given a target word and has to identify the word that preceded it in the spoken sentence. If three responses are correct the task becomes more difficult, for example the target word is not identified until after (instead of before) the sentence has been spoken. Increasing the time between the presentation of the sentence and the point at which the target word is given also makes the task more difficult.

At the end of each session the client is given a score. The audiologist can access the client's data via the manufacturer's website and will therefore know how much time the client has spent in training and any changes that have occurred.

ii) Computer Aided Speech-reading Training (CAST) (Pichora-Fuller and Benguerel, 1991).

CAST was designed for use with pre-retirement adults with mild to moderate hearing loss. It is intended to be completed within ten weeks and covers three basic speechreading skills:

- Visual speech perception
- Linguistic redundancy
- Feedback between conversation partners.

There are eight training sessions and each is focused on a different viseme (sounds that look the same when speechreading).

iii) Conversation Made Easy: Speechreading and Conversation Strategies Training for Adults and Teenagers With Hearing Loss (Tye-Murray, 2002).

'Conversation Made Easy' was designed as different packages for children and for adults and teenagers. The adult and teenager package consist of three sections:

1. *Sounds*: This section is designed to compare and contrast speech sounds that look or sound alike. Every English consonant is included. The listener hears a syllable and is then presented with a number of alternative options on the screen from which they must choose. If their response is incorrect, the syllable is repeated and they try again.

2. *Sentences*: This section is designed for audiovisual training. There are eight exercises of 20 sentences. The listener hears a sentence and then sees four pictures on the screen, from which the best one to illustrate the sentence must be chosen. The focus is on comprehension of the whole

sentence not its component parts. If their response is incorrect, they have the option of selecting from an appropriate clarification strategy, i.e. asking for the sentence to be repeated, simplified, rephrased, for just a key word, or for the sentence to be broken down into two parts.

3. *Everyday situations*: In this section typical communication situations are presented as video clips. In some of the clips, the speaker is making communication more difficult, for example by turning away from the listener while speaking. After watching the clip the listener hears a sentence related to the situation and then see four pictures. Only one of the pictures is directly related to the sentence. If their response is incorrect, they again have the option of selecting from repair strategies but these now also include informing the speaker how to improve communication, for example by looking at the listener whilst speaking.

7.4.3 Speech sounds

Speech is produced in the vocal tract, see *Figure 7.2*. The lungs provide a steady air stream. The vocal cords or folds are open for voiceless sounds and held lightly closed to produce voicing. The vibration of the vocal cords creates a low frequency buzz, known as the fundamental tone, which determines the pitch of the speaker's voice, see *Table 7.3*. The shape of the vocal tract is altered by moving the lips, tongue and other articulators, this alters the resonant characteristics of the vocal tract and causes different sounds or phonemes to be produced.

Table 7.3 *Average frequency of a speaker's fundamental tone*

Speaker	Frequency
Child	260Hz
Female	220Hz
Male	120Hz

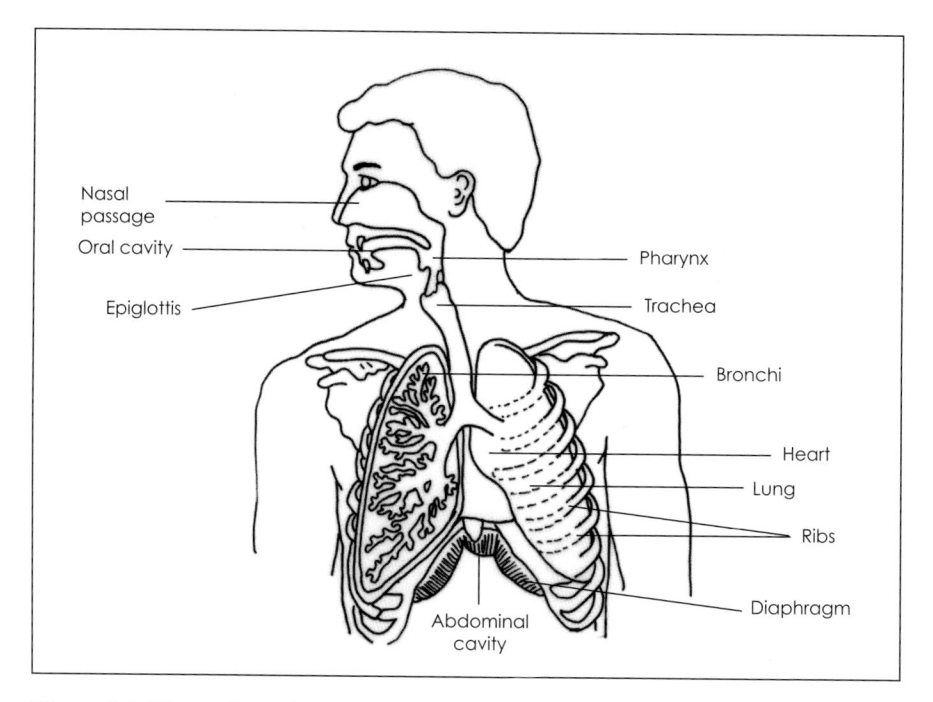

Figure 7.2 *The vocal tract (Reproduced with kind permission of Anglia Distance Learning Ltd)*

i) Vowel recognition

Vowels contain low frequency voicing and also have peaks of energy, called formants, which are created by the resonances in the vocal tract. Vowels are the strongest voiced elements in speech and it is often useful therefore to develop vowel recognition at an

Communication and Auditory Training

early stage in an auditory training programme. Long vowels are the easiest to hear but it is important to realise that hearing a sound does not necessarily mean it can be discriminated from others. The first two vowel formants are important in recognition, see *Figure 7.3*. The second formant is the higher frequency of the two and if the second formant cannot be heard many vowel sounds can be confused. If someone has hearing only up to 2kHz, the second formant (which is important for vowel recognition) will generally not be heard. For example a profoundly deaf person who could hear only first formant information would be likely to confuse 'oo' and 'ee' although they might be able to recognise 'ar'.

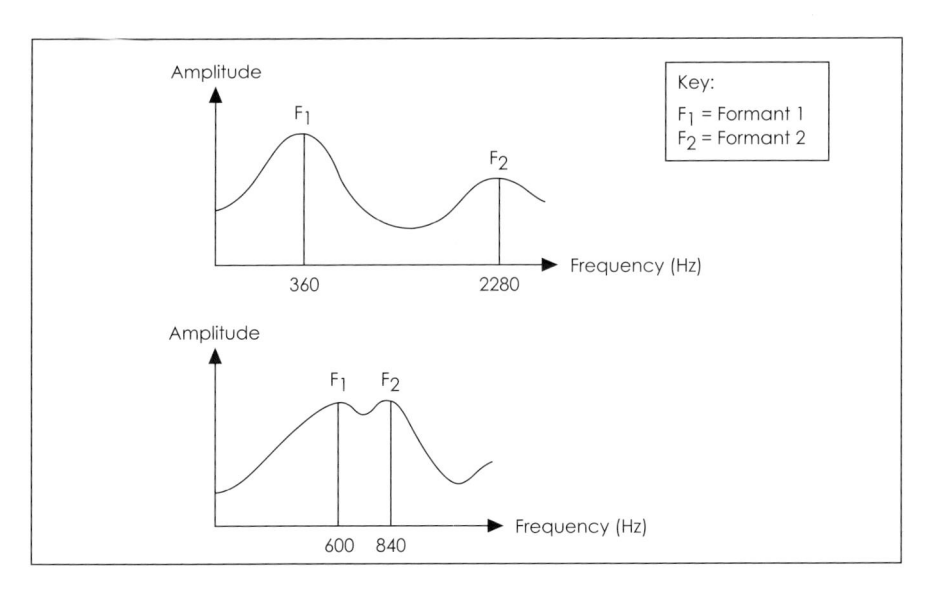

Figure 7.3 Vowel formants

Table 7.4 Examples of some classes of consonants

Consonant class	Examples
Nasals	m,n,ng
Voiced stops/plosives	b,d,g
Voiceless stops/plosives	p,t,k
Voiceless fricatives	f,s,th (as in 'thatch')
Voice fricatives	v,z,th (as in 'that')

ii) Consonant recognition

There are certain consonants that are likely to be confused through hearing alone. Generally most people can distinguish between classes of consonants but within each class confusion is common, see *Table 7.4*. Other errors may occur because a consonant is not heard at all.

Voiced consonants are easier to perceive than voiceless consonants as they include the low frequency sound of voicing which is generally below 400Hz. For example, even with very limited hearing, many deaf people can distinguish between nasal and non-nasal consonants. With severe or profound hearing loss, the different classes of voiced consonants or of voiceless consonants may be confused. For example, voiced stops may be confused with voiced fricatives and voiceless stops may be confused with voiceless fricatives.

The place of articulation is also important in distinguishing consonants but the auditory information that cues these sounds is high frequency and hearing impaired listeners may therefore have trouble in distinguishing front from back sounds, for example the voiced sounds /b/ from /g/ or the voiceless /f/ from /s/.

Communication and Auditory Training

To hear all of the consonant sounds clearly, hearing up to about 6kHz is required. Fricatives are the highest frequency; plosives are generally lower frequency, see *Table 7.5*, but they are very short bursts of sound which are not easy to hear. However, there are useful cues to their recognition available in the silence or *stop* that always precedes a plosive and in the length and transitions of the adjacent vowels.

Table 7.5 Hearing required to recognise plosive sounds

Place of articulation	Phonemes	Frequency
Front	/p/, /b/	800Hz
Mid	/t/, /d/	2kHz
Back	/k/, /g/	4kHz

iii) The audiogram and speech perception of individual sounds

The vowels in speech (*see Figure 7.4*) are relatively low frequency sounds that carry about 90% of the energy in speech. Unfortunately vowels tend to provide the volume of speech rather than the clarity and when the consonants cannot be heard, speech appears to be mumbled and unintelligible. Consonants provide about 90% of the clarity of speech and are therefore needed for speech to be intelligible but they tend to be high in frequency and low in energy. They are therefore more difficult to hear than vowels.

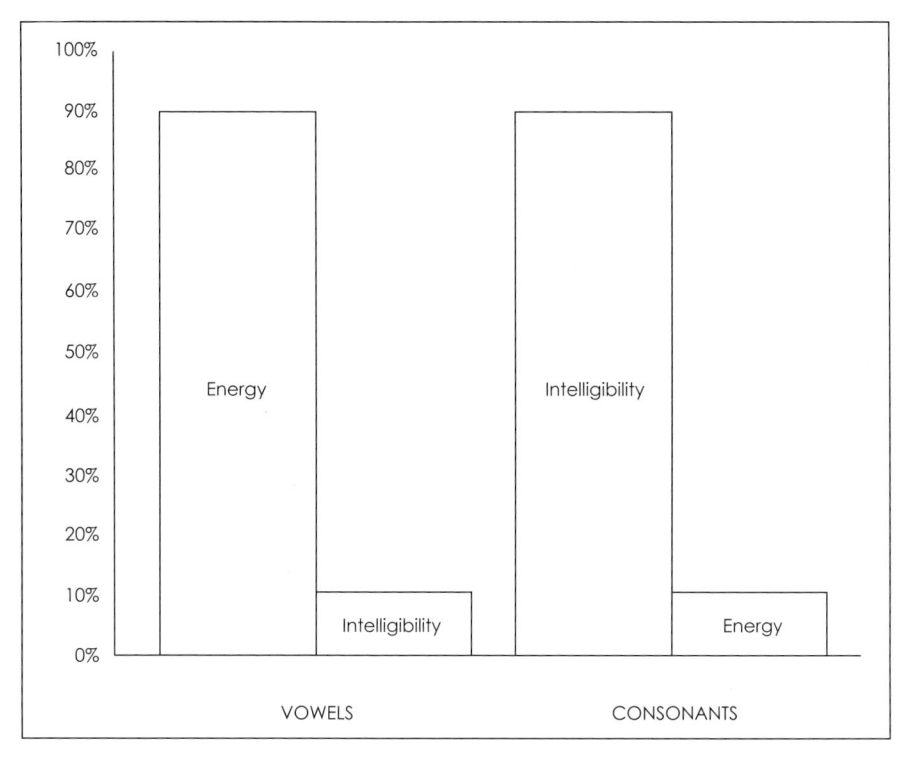

Figure 7.4 *The distribution of energy in speech*

It is possible to make a reasonable prediction from the audiogram of what sounds someone is likely to be able to hear. The 'banana' shape on the audiogram, shown in *Figure 7.5*, indicates the average range and intensity of normal conversational speech. The various phonemes differ in their frequency content and their intensity. Any elements of speech which fall below the person's threshold of hearing will not be heard.

Communication and Auditory Training

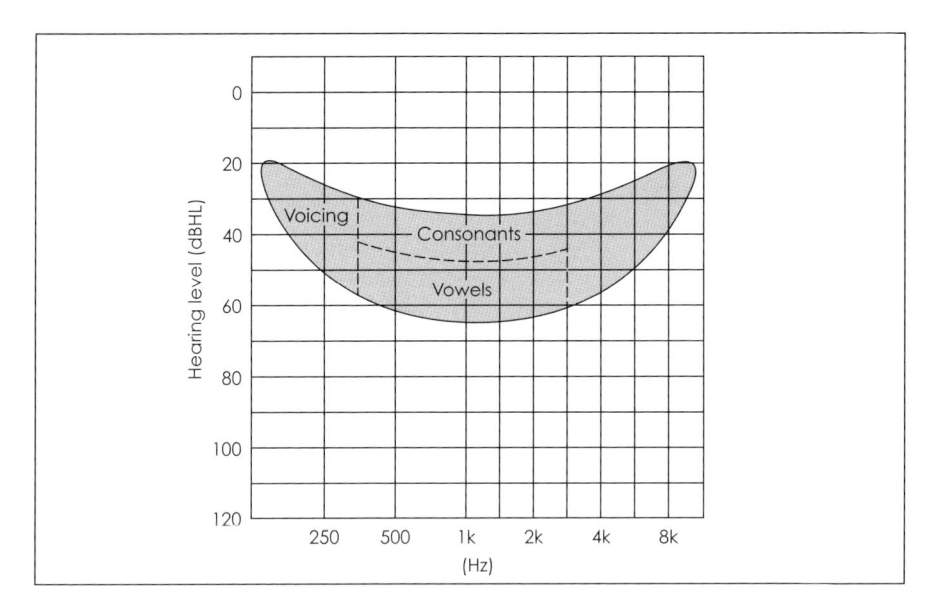

Figure 7.5 An audiogram showing the long term average speech spectrum or 'speech banana' (Reproduced with kind permission of Maltby, 2002)

iv) Sounds in words and sentences

Words and sentences contain many cues apart from individual sounds or phonemes. Words with several syllables are usually easier to understand than single syllable words, although uncommon words or little known terminology are likely to be difficult. With practice, sentences should be easier to comprehend than individual words but complex sentences can still be very difficult.

Many of the cues to length, stress, rhythm, etc. are carried in the low frequency fundamental tone. This information should therefore be available to almost all hearing impaired listeners but some hearing impaired people have poor pitch discrimination and will benefit from training which includes this basic information.

Even when sounds are heard, they are only likely to be understood if they have a meaningful association. Auditory training should therefore revolve around daily situations that the individual may meet in their work, home and social environments.

7.4.4 Lipreading and speech reading

Lipreading is useful with all degrees of hearing impairment. Combining visual information with listening will help to fill the gaps. Although not necessarily realising it, everyone lipreads to some extent when in difficult listening situations, such as in background noise. With a hearing loss, many normal listening situations become difficult and vision becomes increasingly important as an aid to hearing. However, language is predictable to some extent and learning what is possible will help the client to make much better 'guesses' as to what is being said.

A person who lipreads will watch the position of the teeth and lips to add information to their reduced hearing. The lips can, for example, be spread as in /ee/, rounded as in /oo/ or closed as in /m/. Information from lipreading can be useful in discriminating both vowels and consonants although not all sounds look different. Examples of sounds that look the same on the lips (visemes) can be seen in *Table 7.6*.

Table 7.6 Examples of visemes

Visemes		
p	b	m
k	g	ng
ch	j	sh
d	t	n

Training in lipreading includes formal instruction and practice, for example, teaching which phonemes (sounds) and words look alike on the lips and which can be most helpful in making sense of poorly heard speech. Lipreading alone can provide only about 50% of the meaning of speech and becomes very difficult or impossible when the face is hidden. Lipreading is easiest if the speaker is standing about one and a half metres away with the light falling on their face. They should not chew, walk about or speak too fast and it is helpful to practice first with someone who is familiar – and patient!

Most people do not realise that even normally hearing people use lipreading to some extent, especially when in noisy situations. People are usually unaware when they are doing this unless the lip movements and the speech sounds do not match up (e.g. on a film with a faulty sound track) when they may become aware.

Graded practice can help develop lipreading as a highly useful skill which will complement listening with hearing aids. Lipreading is only a part of 'speech reading' which also makes use of information gained from other visual cues such as facial expression, gesture, body position, movement and context, see *Figure 7.6*. It is interesting to note that lipreading, even without sound input, has been shown to activate parts of both the visual and the auditory cortex.

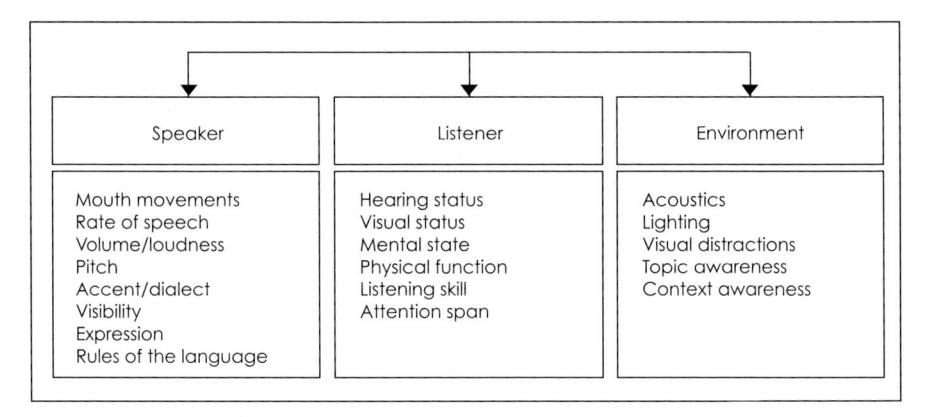

Speaker	Listener	Environment
Mouth movements Rate of speech Volume/loudness Pitch Accent/dialect Visibility Expression Rules of the language	Hearing status Visual status Mental state Physical function Listening skill Attention span	Acoustics Lighting Visual distractions Topic awareness Context awareness

Figure 7.6 Factors that assist or hinder hearing and speech reading

7.5 TELEPHONE TRAINING

Most people use telephones frequently every day although some people, even with normal hearing, are uncomfortable conversing with an unseen person. For most hearing impaired people using the telephone is difficult because only part of the frequency range is available, there are no speech reading cues and the line is not always clear. Some hearing impaired people can communicate well over the phone and need little help but there are others who can only understand if the other person is willing to repeat and rephrase and uses familiar words and simple sentence structures. Amplified handsets may be helpful and hearing aid users may benefit from telephone settings on their aids or from a loop system which can help improve the signal-to-noise ratio. The most severely and profoundly deaf people may have little ability to use the telephone without visible clues and may need to use text or the assistance of another listener perhaps using a speaker phone.

Distinguishing between acoustically similar speech sounds without the aid of lipreading is very difficult. Some of the communication strategies and tactics already introduced will prove useful on the telephone, such as explaining the presence of a hearing loss, asking the speaker to talk slower and reducing any background noise. For example, if it is difficult to recognise who is speaking, it is sensible to ask who it is at the beginning of the call. In general, it is not easy to ensure information has been heard correctly over the telephone and therefore all important details should be double-checked.

Practice on the telephone with familiar people and then with unfamiliar ones will help the client in gaining confidence and communication ability. Exercises should be built up from simple situations to more complex, see *Figure 7.7*, and based on real life needs and situations, for example making a doctor's appointment, talking to a grandchild or asking for help in an emergency.

Conversations on the telephone normally have a very obvious beginning, middle and ending. The beginning is very predictable, and includes saying 'Hello' to the caller, who will normally reply with 'Hello' and then identifying them. The middle of the conversation establishes the purpose of the call and will usually include asking and answering appropriate questions. Each partner in the conversation takes it in turns to speak and the listener is expected to respond appropriately as well as listening. Most telephone conversations are relatively short and about a specific topic, such as making arrangements, obtaining information or making social contact.

If the topic is unknown or changed suddenly, the hearing impaired person is unprepared and may be anxious and unable to follow. If communication breaks down in this way most speakers will try to resolve the situation and the hearing impaired person can suggest strategies that may help. However, not everyone is willing to assist and some people will be embarrassed and prefer to avoid the situation, usually by putting the phone down, if conversation is difficult.

The ending of the conversation is usually very predictable. The caller suggests the conversation should end, such as saying 'I must go' and the other person makes some response in agreement, such as 'See you later then'. Each person says goodbye in turn and this ends the conversation. The rules of conversation are such that they can be used to help the hearing impaired person to anticipate and to manage most telephone conversations.

Communication and Auditory Training 147

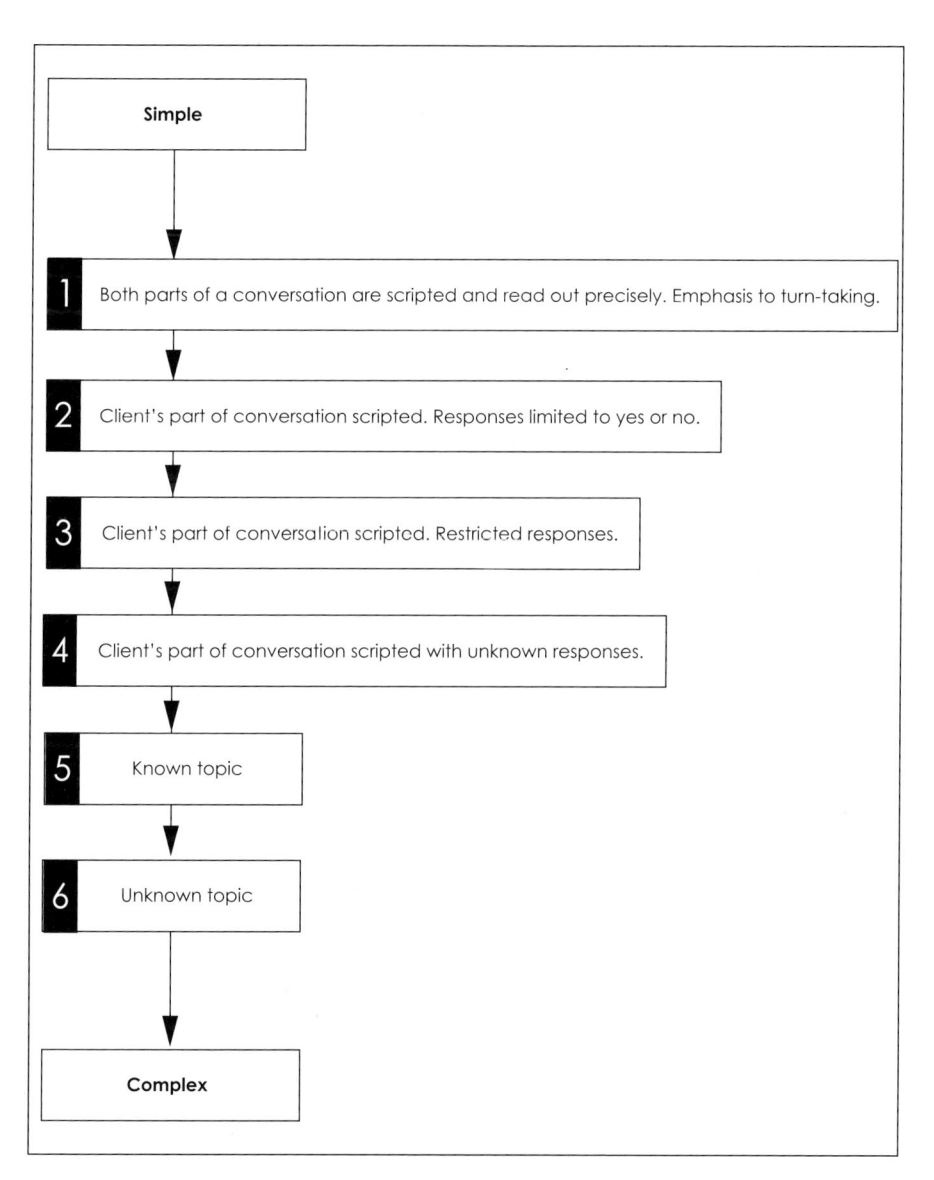

Simple

1. Both parts of a conversation are scripted and read out precisely. Emphasis to turn-taking.

2. Client's part of conversation scripted. Responses limited to yes or no.

3. Client's part of conversation scripted. Restricted responses.

4. Client's part of conversation scripted with unknown responses.

5. Known topic

6. Unknown topic

Complex

Figure 7.7 A flow chart of graded telephone conversation exercises

7.6 SPEECH CONSERVATION

Most sensorineural hearing loss develops slowly and gradually and for some time the individual adjusts without even noticing. A sudden hearing loss will have a much greater effect on hearing ability and speech production as there has been no opportunity to adjust. A severe sudden loss is likely to affect speech due to the sudden loss of auditory feedback.

Where a sudden, total hearing loss occurs in adulthood, speech conservation is a major factor. This will require special coaching and the services of a skilled speech and language therapist to teach the person to monitor and modify their speech not by the sound of their voice (although they will, of course, use any residual hearing they may have) but by the feel of the speech organs in motion and the positional sense of lips and tongue against the teeth and hard palate.

Longstanding hearing loss, especially if severe or profound, will usually result in deteriorating speech articulation as the memory of how to produce clear speech fades without the auditory feedback.

Chapter 8
Counselling

8.1 WHAT IS COUNSELLING?

A definition of counselling from the Oxford English Dictionary is:

The process of assisting or guiding clients, especially by a trained person on a professional basis, to resolve especially personal, social, or psychological problems and difficulties (Allen, 1991).

Counselling skills are based on normal communication skills, see *Table 8.1*. Counselling is a part of the rehabilitation process and widely used in Rehabilitative Audiology. There are two types of counselling:

1. *Personal-adjustment counselling* is client-centred and concerned with empowering clients, by exploring their feelings and attitudes. It includes helping clients to come to terms with their hearing loss, helping them overcome difficulties and referring them on where necessary.

2. *Informational counselling* is directive and concerned with giving advice and information or with acting on the client's behalf. It involves making sure clients understand all about their hearing loss, treatment options that are available and how the loss may affect their life. It includes

talking through the use of hearing aids, helping clients to overcome difficulties with their hearing aids and assisting them to develop the skills needed to deal with the hearing loss effectively.

Table 8.1 Counselling skills are heavily dependent on normal communication skills

Communication skill	Counselling skill
Understanding	Ensuring clients understand all about their hearing loss, its effect and treatment options available. How to fit, use and care for their hearing aids.
Talking	Helping clients to come to terms with their hearing loss and talking through use of the hearing aids.
Listening	Assisting clients to develop their communication skills in order to deal with their hearing loss most effectively.

8.2 STRESS

Loss of hearing may affect roles, opportunities and activities. Social situations are difficult and often result in confusion, frustration, disappointment and anger, frequently heightened by a lack of understanding from others. The stress may be such that the deaf person begins to withdraw from social situations and avoidance behaviour is often the start of a downward spiral in which situations that are unavoidable become increasingly stressful and feared.

A small degree of stress is usually seen as being positive. We tend to work harder and better if the situation is a little stressful.

However, there is a fine line between positive and negative degrees of stress. Stress and panic can be debilitating and result in such sympathetic nervous system reactions as increased blood pressure, increased pulse rate and sweating. Too much stress should be viewed as a warning and an indication of a need to change.

Stress is a very usual reaction to hearing loss. Too much stress is generally due to a perception of lack of control. Stress management aims to give a sense of control over the variables that are contributing to the stress. Feeling able to exert control, even from time-to-time, reduces stress. Many variables, apart from the hearing loss itself, can increase hearing difficulty and stress but there are very few situations where some degree of control is not possible. Extra effort is generally involved to improve the listening situation and, for this to occur, the situation has to be considered sufficiently important to merit the effort. Counselling can help the individual to come to terms with their hearing loss and provide strategies to modify behaviour and/or the environment in order to reduce stress. Counselling is therefore a central and indispensable part of Rehabilitative Audiology.

Assertiveness is also an important skill that can help in overcoming stress by taking control in facilitating communication. Asking others to speak louder or to repeat, seeking clarification or attempting to modify the environment to provide better listening conditions all involve the need for the client to be assertive. Unfortunately, when under stress, it is easy to become passive or aggressive.

- *Passive behaviour* (shyness, nervousness, helplessness, fear, etc.) can prevent the individual from expressing their needs or emotions effectively and make them unable to stand up for their rights.

- *Aggressive behaviour* may allow them to stand up for their rights but only in a way that is domineering, intimidating, objectionable and rude.

- *Assertive behaviour* is confident but considerate and calm. It allows needs and emotions to be expressed honestly and directly but in an appropriate manner. Assertive behaviour is often essential to success.

8.3 THE RATIONALE OF COUNSELLING

The basic rationale behind counselling is based on six principles:

1. People are capable of change.
2. Behaviours that are harmful, limiting or generally undesirable warrant change.
3. Techniques and intervention, such as instruction, support, advice, encouragement and persuasion, can assist change.
4. Clients who seek counselling do need help.
5. Clients believe change is possible.
6. Clients will take an active role in change management.

Counselling is designed to help people resolve their problems and can be used to help the individual to accept hearing loss and to achieve realistic goals. A successful professional relationship with the client has to be developed and, in order to facilitate this, counselling should be carried out somewhere private and comfortable. The counselling process begins by obtaining information and assessing the client's needs so that realistic goals can be agreed. The audiologist should always respond openly and honestly to the client's questions but should be aware that there may be needs that are hidden behind the client's comments and questions. The client will often leave things out or over-generalise, saying for example "I don't understand *anyone*" or "*Everyone* shouts at me". The counsellor needs to question these assumptions in order to reach below the surface and clarify the client's true objectives.

The aim of counselling is to help the client to develop a positive approach and make practical changes but it can only be productive if emotions are recognised and worked through.

8.4 COUNSELLING SKILLS

Counselling is concerned with helping someone through a difficult time. The skills needed for counselling are those that are involved in all successful social interactions. Counselling does not have to be carried out by a professional counsellor. Non-professional counsellors, such as friends, family, clergy, teachers and lawyers may all be involved in informal counselling from time-to-time. Indeed, most people are capable of becoming effective counsellors if they are genuinely interested in people and want to help. Some people will be 'natural' counsellors but, for others, counselling skills can be developed through knowledge, practice and experience.

What makes a good counsellor? The person undertaking this role should be well-adjusted, have a positive attitude, be non-judgemental, knowledgeable and a good listener; they should show empathy and respect. The relationship between the client and the counsellor is therefore critical and is usually the most important single variable in the rehabilitation process.

An individual approach is needed to suit each particular counselling relationship. Whatever the approach, it must be carried out in an atmosphere of unconditional positive regard, in other words with genuineness, warmth, respect and empathy. The counsellor needs to be aware of how their responses may impact on the client. Both verbal cues (such as tone of voice and rate of utterance) and non-verbal cues (such as body posture, gesture, physical closeness, facial expression and eye contact) are important and the counsellor should be aware of these so that they do not appear uninterested, critical or insincere. Undertaking counselling in a quiet, comfortable, private place, restating the content of what the client says and reflecting back their expressed feelings can all help promote an atmosphere of empathy.

The following counselling skills are the main ones that an audiologist will need to use in the rehabilitation process and which need to be developed and practised. However, to use them successfully, the audiologist must also know when and where to use them:

- Empathy and understanding
- Patience and tact
- Unconditional regard
- Appropriate verbal and non-verbal communication skills
- An ability to ask open questions
- Challenging beliefs
- Excellent listening skills
- An ability to give simple but appropriate explanations
- An appreciation of when it is necessary to refer on.

8.5 THE AUDIOLOGIST AS A COUNSELLOR

8.5.1 Professional behaviour

The behaviour of the professional provides the framework for the client-counsellor relationship. Professional behaviours used will depend on the circumstances but can generally be seen to fall into one of the following models. The professional will use one or a mixture of these models of behaviour, possibly without realising how they are behaving. However, an awareness of one's behaviour as a professional is important if counselling skills are to be improved.

- *The expert model* is where the counsellor takes on the role of the expert who 'knows best' and will control the situation and make all the decisions, see *Figure 8.1*. The expert may not necessarily explore the client's whole situation nor necessarily explain things fully so that the client can make their own decisions.

- *The transplant model* is one in which the professional is still seen as the expert who controls the situation, selects which hearing aids are appropriate and sets the objectives for rehabilitation. However, the client is empowered by the expert as they provide the client with necessary knowledge and skills.

- *The consumer model* views the client as having the right to choose what they want. The audiologist will listen and try to understand the client's situation and views so that they can provide appropriate options and knowledge to enable the client to come to their own realistic and informed choices. This model is a true partnership but involves more time and resources than either of the other models.

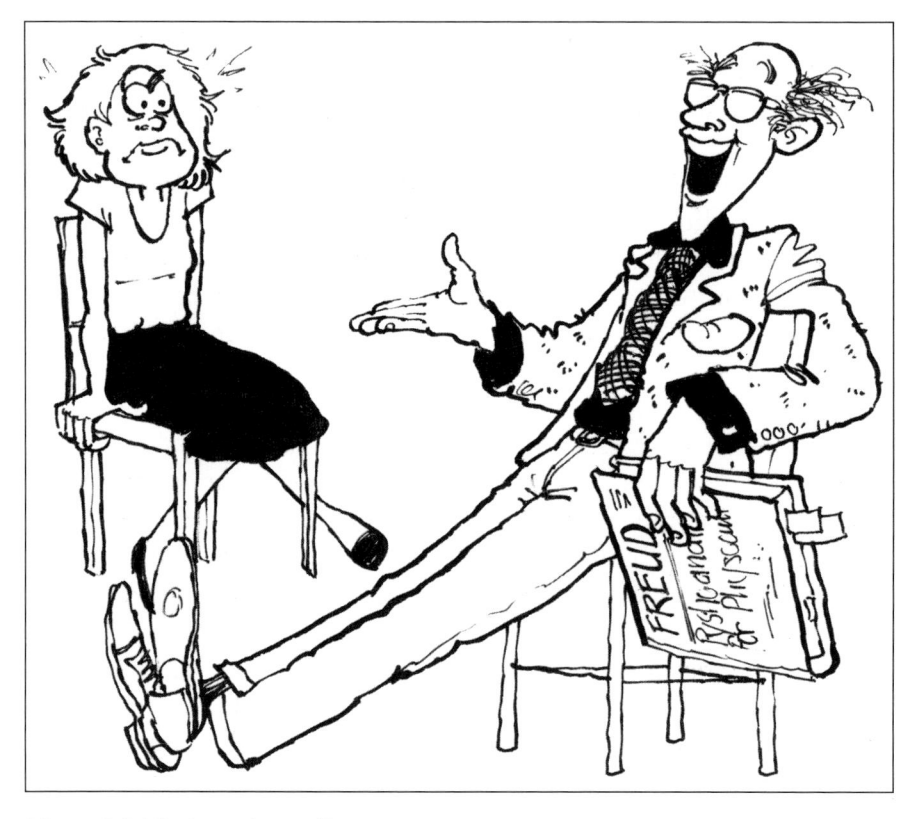

Figure 8.1 *The 'expert' counsellor*

Most audiologists will use different models at different times to meet the needs of their clients. A flexible approach that treats the client as an individual with particular needs and that shares information and skills in an atmosphere of warmth and respect will generally result in the best outcomes.

8.5.2 Counselling in Audiology

Counselling is an integral part of the role of an audiologist involved with hearing aid fitting. Counselling occurs in every hearing aid dispensing. However, it may be intentional or unintentional and many audiologists do not develop an organised approach or are uncertain what the limits of their counselling should be.

It is natural to introduce counselling into the audiometric situation. Audiologists have a good understanding of hearing impairment and the difficulties it creates and are therefore in an ideal position to counsel hearing impaired individuals. Counselling is likely to be most successful if it is intentional, planned and underpinned by knowledge of counselling theory and techniques. The course of adjustment to hearing loss is unpredictable and there are many different counselling approaches which can be used separately or together to suit the individual and their circumstances. Counselling approaches used in Rehabilitative Audiology tend to be based largely on experiential theory, behavioural theory and cognitive theory:

- An *experiential* (client-centred) approach is non-directive, that is it does not recommend or guide in an authoritarian manner but helps the client to take responsibility for their own progress and helps them to build up the acceptance and self awareness they need to do this.

- A *behavioural* approach is directive and uses positive reinforcement, whilst guiding the client through successive stages, towards the desired goal.

- A *cognitive* approach is one that disputes negative views, and questions any stated assumptions that could stand in the way of successful counselling.

The role of an audiologist-counsellor is to respond to individual needs and provide short-term support to help the client adjust to the communication difficulties associated with hearing loss. In general this will involve:

- Problem identification
- Informational counselling
- Challenging beliefs
- Goal setting
- Support
- Problem-solving strategies.

8.6 EFFECTIVE COUNSELLING

8.6.1 Problem identification

The first step in the rehabilitative process is problem identification. In order to find the solutions to problems, it is first necessary to identify the problems. Hearing aids do not give back normal hearing and the degree of help derived from amplification varies widely between individuals. Problem identification involves ascertaining the extent and nature of the hearing loss and its impact on the individual's life. Problem identification is a theme that runs throughout the rehabilitation process and which starts when the client first enters the clinic.

Although, in audiology, the case history is the first main fact-finding exercise, communication and adjustment difficulties are also assessed, through the hearing test, through discussion and through questionnaires. Many factors may be important in the rehabilitation process and a wide range of factors must therefore be investigated in addition to hearing levels, for example:

- Personality
- Support from family/friends
- Professional support
- Cause of hearing loss

- Rate of onset
- Age
- Gender
- Work/leisure activities
- Communication environments
- Family situation
- Life experiences
- Additional disabilities
- Expectations
- Motivation
- Attitude to hearing aids
- Level of understanding.

Intervention should be needs-based and success measured by how far needs and expectations are met.

8.6.2 Informational counselling

It is much easier to accept a problem if it is understood. Informational counselling is therefore essential and integral to the whole process of rehabilitation. Informational counselling will not only involve teaching but also dialogue and working through emotions, feelings and attitudes so that the client can understand the impact of hearing loss.

Informational counselling should be related to the client, their hearing loss, their situation and their needs. It will necessarily involve a sensitive explanation of the hearing loss and its effects, and of hearing aids and what these can and cannot do for the client. It will usually include a discussion around different types of hearing aids and how they work, in order that the client will be enabled to make a hearing aid selection based on knowledge and understanding. Later, informational counselling will include such things as how to take care of the aid, how to troubleshoot problems and what help may be available from assistive listening devices.

Counselling the partner or family is also important as they too need to understand the problems. Their support is often vital to a successful outcome. Sometimes playing a recording simulating a hearing loss can be very helpful as, without the experience, it is difficult to appreciate how someone can 'hear' but not understand. The supportive others also need to know how to recognise when listening conditions are poor and what they can do to improve them.

8.6.3 Motivation and challenging beliefs

Motivation is self-directed behaviour and is critical to achieving successful change. For optimum motivation (Kemp, 1988) the client must know what they want (have goals), believe them possible and be able to obtain meaningful rewards with minimal associated 'costs'. Costs may be financial or related to time or they may be psychological and relate to self-esteem or emotional discomfort. The benefits must outweigh the costs if the client is to be motivated. If behaviour is associated with positive feedback or reward it will be reinforced and maintained but a client who is self-motivated is far more likely to succeed with hearing aids than anyone who feels pushed into the decision by a family member or friend.

The individual's beliefs and attitudes, as well as their motivation, will be related to their goals. In order to understand the client's beliefs and attitudes, the audiologist needs to understand the client's situation, their personality and their view of the future. It is important that the client believes they are capable of success. Any negative beliefs have to be challenged, for example:

'How do you know...?'
'What is the worst thing that could happen if...?', or
'How can I convince you that...?'

Acceptance of the hearing loss and its effects is a necessary first step. Many people will try to hide their problems, often due to embarrassment and fear of appearing stupid but, in reality, waiting until obvious communication errors have occurred is much more likely to lead the listener to make unfortunate assumptions about the listener's intelligence.

8.6.4 Goal setting

Rehabilitation should be structured and goal-directed. It is our goals that tend to initiate behaviour and to guide the outcome. The basic goal of rehabilitation is to narrow the gap between the current situation and 'normal' communication by various means, usually including enhancing hearing ability through wearing hearing aids and/or using assistive devices and by using strategies or tactics to reduce the demands of the environment.

If the rehabilitation process is to be successful, the client's goals must be realistic, so time spent at an early stage adjusting expectations is time well spent. The client and significant others need to understand that hearing aids do not give back normal hearing and, however advanced they are, they are still only aids to hearing. There will still be difficult listening situations. Visual information, context, etc. will still be needed to support hearing.

A client is very unlikely to succeed with their goals if depression and other negative emotions are not faced and self esteem improved. Support to achieve this may be in the form of emotional support, stress management, assertiveness training and problem solving. One of the objectives of the audiologist-counsellor is to provide emotional support so that the client will feel able to explore their feelings.

8.6.5 Problem-solving strategies

Successful communication is dependent on the listener, the speaker, the environment and the message. Unfortunately, some clients will have developed negative strategies which need to be unlearned. These may include fearing conversation, withdrawing from social contact or becoming angry and aggressive, self-pitying or helpless. A client with a hearing loss (particularly those with a long-standing loss) may need help to develop positive communication strategies and to re-learn to listen. Hearing aids can improve hearing but listening is an *active* process that involves attention and effort. Strategies that can be learned to help improve communication may be facilitative or repairing:

i) Facilitative strategies

Facilitative strategies manipulate the environment in order to improve communication success. There are many relatively simple strategies, such as avoiding talking in noisy places, moving as far away from noise sources as possible, using carpets, soft furnishings and table cloths, etc. to reduce noise, and rearranging furniture and lighting to give the listener the best possible position for listening and lipreading.

Instructional strategies can also be very helpful, for example asking the speaker to:

- Stand about a metre away
- Face the listener
- Ensure the speaker's face is visible
- Ensure light falls on the speaker's face and not in the listener's eyes
- Obtain the listener's attention before they speak

- Speak a little slower and a little louder
- Pause at the end of sentences
- Use non-verbal cues such as facial expression and gesture
- Write down key words
- Respond to requests for repetition or clarification
- Ask the listener to repeat the message to ensure that it has been understood correctly.

ii) Repairing strategies

When communication breaks down the listener has a choice to make, they can withdraw from the conversation, ignore the breakdown, pretend that they have understood or call on repair strategies. Pretence or ignoring may be used because the listener does not want to disrupt the conversation or to let the speaker know they are having a problem, or it may be because they lack the skills or are unwilling to make the effort required. Non-specific repair structures, for example saying 'What?' or 'Pardon?', are very common and will usually result in repetition of what was said, but unfortunately frequent repetition of 'What?' can be very irritating.

Specific repair strategies usually require assertiveness on the part of the client and a willingness to help on the part of the speaker. For example if the listener asks the speaker to repeat or rephrase what they have said, the strategy can only be successful if the speaker does so. Different strategies may be used at different times but, in general, specific strategies, such as asking for the message to be rephrased, simplified or confirmed tend to be most successful. This is despite the fact that they can be more disruptive of the conversation.

The speaker can benefit from specific suggestions as to how they can improve the communication process. This will usually include explaining that the listener does have a hearing loss and what would be helpful, such as slightly slower speech.

WATCH (Montgomery, 1994) is an acronym that provides a useful and simple method for clients to remember strategies that will enhance the communication experience:

W: Watch the speaker's mouth not their eyes.
The importance of facial expression, gesture and intonation should be stressed and strategies can be taught that will help speech recognition.

A: Ask specific questions.
How to ask questions is an important skill to be learned. The communication partner should also be requested to repeat, rephrase or add helpful information to the message.

T: Tell about your hearing loss.
Informing others that there is a problem and giving brief instruction on how they can help, for example 'I have a hearing loss, please could you talk a little more slowly and make sure you are facing me when you are speaking.'

C: Change the environment so it is free of distractions including excessive background noise.
At home or in other familiar situations, this could involve moving furniture to improve access to auditory and visual cues, using a tablecloth to reduce noise at mealtimes, etc.

H: Hearing health care knowledge should be acquired.
This includes information about hearing, hearing aids and assistive devices and about local and other resources.

8.7 REFERRAL

There will be times when the client needs more counselling than the audiologist can give and when a counselling referral is therefore needed. If the client cannot move forward, continues to experience depression or other negative emotions, has persistent unrealistic expectations or underlying issues that are difficult or impossible to resolve, the situation may be beyond the competence of the audiologist or may require more intensive and longer term support than they are able to provide. In some cases, it may be the client's partner or a family member who holds persistent unrealistic expectations or who is intolerant of the communication problems.

In order to be able to react appropriately, the audiologist needs to have knowledge of local counselling and other mental health care services in the area. It is also helpful to know if any of these are familiar with hearing problems.

When explaining the need for onward referral to the client, the audiologist should try to be honest and straightforward and help the client to appreciate that their problems are very real and their need for help is similar to many other people in the same situation.

Chapter 9
Anxiety, Depression and Therapy

9.1 ANXIETY

9.1.1 Anxiety defined

Anxiety is a mood state characterised by negative effect, body tension and apprehension (American Psychiatric Association, 1994). Anxiety is an essential part of survival, for instance the fear reaction allows the body to mobilise the energy needed to flee from danger. Thus anxiety clearly has evolutionary value. In moderation anxiety is good for us as it increases vigilance and concentration. However anxiety can be viewed as a response on a continuum with too little or too much being detrimental and with extreme anxiety having a destructive effect on everyday life. At its most extreme irrational anxiety can become an anxiety disorder. Anxiety disorders are characterised by intense dread, nervousness or fear, which may be experienced in response to a particular situation or event, or in anticipation of an anxiety causing event. A feeling of lack of control may be accompanied by physical symptoms, such as sweating and rapid breathing and heart rate. To be recognised as a clinical disorder, the symptoms must interfere with everyday life and be long-standing (generally over at least six months). Clinical anxiety disorders may be classified as:

- *Generalised anxiety disorders*: excessive indiscriminating worry leading to restlessness, sleep disturbance, irritability and muscle tension all of which is unproductive.

Approximately 4% of the population suffer from generalised anxiety disorder.

- *Panic disorders*: severe unexpected panic attacks in which the individual feels out of control. The attack must involve at least four of the following symptoms to be clinically defined as a panic attack: chest pain, sweating, dizziness, nausea and a feeling of choking. The individual fears and avoids places in which they would feel unsafe if they experienced a panic attack. This can develop into agoraphobia, which is a fear of open spaces.

- *Social phobia*: Intense persistent fear of social situations to the extent where it disrupts everyday life and causes great distress. Typical situations would be eating in restaurants or attending parties in which the individual may fear humiliation. Such anxiety is often accompanied by avoidance behaviour and is very common amongst the hearing impaired.

9.1.2 Models of anxiety

Personality may be based on levels of cortical arousal (Eysenck, 1967). Extroverts are those with low levels of cortical arousal who therefore seek out risks. Introverts or neurotics have a high level of cortical arousal and therefore avoid risky or arousing situations. Anxious individuals are thought to have high levels of cortical arousal and autonomous nervous system activity. Irrational anxiety has its basis in a faulty processing of reality where people tend to overestimate danger and underestimate their ability to cope.

Conditioning theory provides a logical explanation for 'irrational' fears:

1. *Classical conditioning* occurs when a certain response becomes associated or paired with a particular stimulus. For example, an individual may have felt anxious when involved in a particular social event. The individual may then strongly associate anxiety with all social events and thereafter become extremely anxious at the suggestion of any social activity. The anxiety has become a conditioned response to social activity.

2. *Operant conditioning* occurs when the individual is instrumental in determining the consequences of an action. For example, the individual who has experienced anxiety as a result of a particular social activity may learn that avoidance of social activity may reduce the fear. Avoidance behaviour produces feelings of security as the feared situation is avoided but in fact this reinforces and maintains the fear.

Cognitive theorists suggest that the way an individual appraises a situation determines their reaction to it. If they appraise it in a negative way they are likely to develop a fear response. Negative appraisal involves seeing a situation as a high threat and as being unable to cope with it (Beck 1985). Low self confidence and negative thinking are seen as key factors in negative appraisal. The thinking process (cognition) is the primary factor in maintaining anxiety.

Using a psychodynamic model, extreme anxiety may occur when unconscious internal conflicts are triggered by association with external demands. In his work on anxiety, Freud (1926) claimed one of the functions of anxiety is to warn of danger and therefore to trigger higher psychological defence mechanisms. Defence mechanisms may, however, be maladaptive.

9.1.3 Treatment for anxiety

Behavioural therapy is based on changing behaviour. It assumes that maladaptive behaviour patterns have been learned and the aim of therapy is that these should be unlearned. In theory, behavioural therapy uses classical conditioning, whilst behaviour modification is based on operant conditioning. In practice there is considerable overlap. Methods of behavioural therapy that may be used include relaxation and prolonged experience:

- *Systematic desensitisation* is where the client is taught to relax in the presence of anxiety provoking stimuli. Progressive muscle relaxation is taught initially in imagined situations. A positive stimulus, such as eating, is sometimes paired with a feared stimulus to increase relaxation.

- *Flooding* is prolonged experience of the feared stimulus, which is sometimes used to prevent avoidance behaviour usually supported by cognitive therapy to reduce distortions of thinking and perception.

Cognitive therapy involves cognitive restructuring. This focuses on negative thinking and attempts to shift it to a more positive and realistic representation of the situation. The client is taught about anxiety and their fear of failure is challenged. They may be asked, for example, to list their fears and be encouraged to test the validity and probability of them arising. In general, graded activities are used to build up more positive responses.

Individuals who are highly socially anxious tend to expend effort in planning ways to avoid stressful situations or to conceal their anxiety rather than in attempting to face and improve the situation (Vassilopoulos, 2008). Depression is a common outcome and anxiety linked with depression is more common than anxiety alone.

The aim of psychodynamic therapy, see *Figure 9.1*, is to reach beneath a person's anxiety to hidden feelings and conflict, which are usually traced back to the past and are often in relation to a parent. The therapist interprets what might be beneath the anxiety and then works through the hidden feelings to reduce the anxiety symptoms and tries to teach the client more positive defence mechanisms.

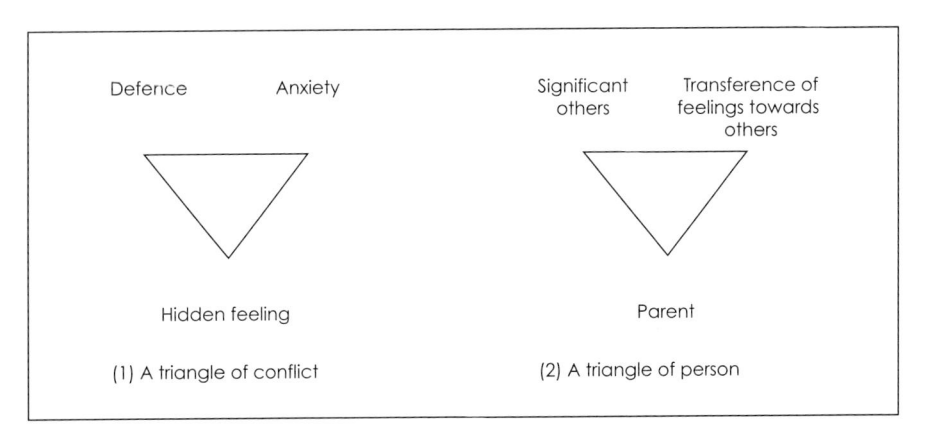

```
   Defence        Anxiety           Significant      Transference of
                                      others         feelings towards
                                                          others

         \      /                          \      /
          \    /                            \    /
           \  /                              \  /
            \/                                \/

       Hidden feeling                       Parent

    (1) A triangle of conflict         (2) A triangle of person
```

Figure 9.1 *A triangle model of therapy*

9.2 DEPRESSION

9.2.1 Depression defined

Everyone experiences low mood from time-to-time. Depression, in response to a loss, including loss of hearing, is a normal response. It is only when depression begins to disrupt all areas of a person's life, so that he or she cannot work or maintain relationships, that it is considered clinical.

Clinical depression is difficult to distinguish from deep unhappiness and is viewed by many as simply the end of a continuum. People who are diagnosed as having clinical depression have a much higher risk of suicide than the general population (Paykel, 1989; Botswik and Pankratz, 2000). The audiologist is not trained to diagnose or treat clinical depression and must refer on any clients who may be clinically depressed.

Depressed mood is a prerequisite for a diagnosis of depression but other symptoms may include:

- Sleep disturbance
- Increased or decreased appetite
- Excessive tiredness
- Decrease in sexual interest
- Slowed thinking
- Feelings of shame, guilt and self-disgust
- Suicidal thoughts
- Particularly low mood in the mornings.

Depression is one of the commonest adult psychological problems. It is estimated that between 3% and 7% of the general population suffer clinically significant depression (Paykel, 1989). Depression related to the onset of hearing loss is understandably prevalent.

9.2.2 Approaches to treating depression

The work of Aaron Beck (1972, 1995) has been influential in recent developments in cognitive models of treating depression. His approach regards the main causal factor as a disorder of cognition. Beck regards the depressive person's thinking as

Anxiety, Depression and Therapy

excessively negative, with the individual viewing themselves, the world and the future in a negative way. His theory proposes that in the course of their development people gather knowledge about themselves and the world which is stored as 'schema'. These schema form beliefs and assumptions that serve as the basic structures a person uses to perceive, understand and think about the world. The schema of a depressed person are generated in a way that results in a negative bias when interpreting experiences and in negative automatic thoughts which cause depressed mood, see *Figure 9.2*.

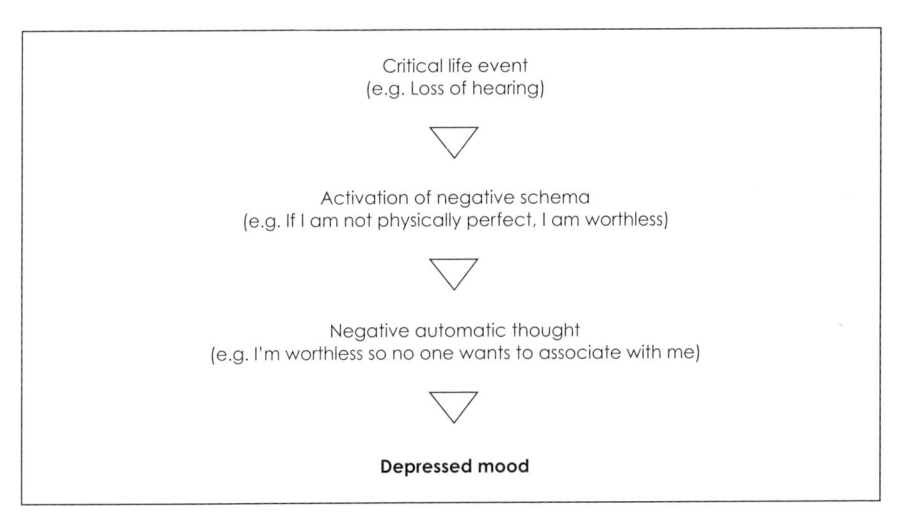

```
            Critical life event
            (e.g. Loss of hearing)
                    ▽

         Activation of negative schema
  (e.g. If I am not physically perfect, I am worthless)
                    ▽

          Negative automatic thought
 (e.g. I'm worthless so no one wants to associate with me)
                    ▽

              Depressed mood
```

Figure 9.2 Development of depressed mood

Negative biases can influence the generation of negative thoughts (Field, 2000), for example:

- *Arbitrary inference*: for example my friend is not answering the phone so she must be avoiding me.
- *Selective abstraction*: that is ignoring positive signals

and concentrating only on occasional negative signals, for example my friend says they would like to visit but they are busy for the next few days therefore they must not want to see me.

- *Overgeneralisation of negative occurrences*: for example after a misunderstanding leads to an argument, I think everyone hates me.
- *Personalisation*: that is seeing everything as relating to oneself, for example if people are bored I assume it is my fault.
- *Magnification* of negative events.
- *Dichotomous thoughts*: that is very 'black and white', for example, without hearing I can't do anything.
- *Unreasonable demands*: for example, I should be able to communicate at a social occasion without difficulty.

Cognitive therapy has four main components:

1. *Education*: during which individuals receive information about depression and the therapy they are going to receive.
2. *Goal setting and graded activities*: Many depressed people withdraw from their normal activities, which tends to maintain the depressive state. One of the key strategies in cognitive therapy is identifying these activities and setting graded activities, together with homework to be carried out between sessions.
3. *Identification of negative thoughts*: The depressed person is helped to identify the negative thoughts that are involved with how they feel. These may be discovered through role play in clinical sessions or through the individual keeping a diary of thoughts, feelings and experiences.

Anxiety, Depression and Therapy

4. *Challenging*: Once the negative thoughts have been identified, the client is encouraged to challenge them and test their validity. In depression these core beliefs tend to centre around the need to be loved and to do well in all situations at all costs. The client tends to have a negative view of themselves, the world and the future based on biased past experiences. The difficulty for the therapist is to disentangle the real from the imagined failures and enable the client to form a more balanced view about themselves and the future.

Other approaches that may also be used include behavioural, psychodynamic and biological:

- The *behavioural approach* views depression and helplessness as learned through lack of reinforcement or reward for psychologically healthy behaviour.
- The *psychodynamic approach* places great emphasis on the unconscious which prevents painful or unacceptable thoughts from entering consciousness. The root of such thoughts is usually seen as occurring in childhood. On the whole psychodynamic therapies are time-consuming, expensive and ineffective. However, non-directive interpersonal therapy, where the client is allowed to talk freely and direct therapy sessions, can be effective and the client often gains insight into their behaviour.
- The *biological approach* uses medication to treat depression. Sometimes drugs are needed to move the client to a stage where they can participate in therapy. However antidepressants are not effective for all clients and can cause side effects. They tend to be most effective when combined with therapy to change thinking patterns.

Cognitive therapy is generally more effective than behavioural change (Dobson, 2001) which focuses *only* on changing behaviour and not on the thinking behind it. Behavioural therapy is therefore commonly used in conjunction with cognitive therapies in what is known as *Cognitive Behavioural Therapy* (CBT). CBT challenges the underlying problems involved in depression and teaches coping skills. Clients are encouraged to engage in rewarding experiences through which the desired behaviours can be reinforced.

9.3 NEUROLINGUISTIC PROGRAMMING

9.3.1 Development of NLP

Neurolinguistic programming (NLP) was developed from psychotherapy by Richard Bandler and John Grinder in the 1970s (Bandler and Grinder, 1979). They based their methodology on observations of communication strategies used by Fritz Perls, Virginia Satir and Milton Erickson who were highly successful psychotherapists of that time. All were found to imitate or respond to their client's movements and amongst the strategies noted were:

- Maintaining eye contact
- Matching predicates (verbs, adverbs, and adjectives) to those used by the client
- Matching body language (posture, gesture, etc.) to that of the client
- Matching the breathing rhythm of the client.

When using NLP, instead of attending only to the words that are spoken, the person's whole behaviour is observed including both verbal and non-verbal cues. This information is then used with the overall aim of invoking personal changes to help the client overcome their life problems. In the methodology, this is assumed possible because it is considered that:

1. Individuals do not see the real world but use an individual set of beliefs to filter reality. It is this filtered reality that people act upon not reality itself.

2. Life and the mind are systems and therefore any change will have consequences on the system as a whole.

A practitioner who uses NLP will note the unconscious signs that people make, such as gestures, eye movements, facial movements, breathing, voice tone and the use of certain parts of speech (predicates), and respond to these. These external visual, auditory and kinaesthetic cues are said to represent problems, desires, feelings, beliefs and outcomes, examples are given in *Figure 9.3* and *Table 9.1*. The methodology is based on an acceptance that:

- There is a positive intention to every behaviour, even those which appear on the surface to be totally negative.
- Every behaviour communicates according to the response it produces and not necessarily what was intended.
- Choice is better than no choice and multiple descriptions are better than one.
- The most flexible element in a system is the one that will have the most influence.
- People have all the internal resources they need to succeed.
- Failure is not an option but feedback can be obtained.

Table 9.1 Examples of verbs that are said to provide sensory cues to the type of internal mental process being used

Sensory processing	Verb	Example
Visual	See	I can see that
	Appears	That appears correct
Kinaesthetic	Grasp	I can grasp that
	Feels	That feels right
Auditory	Rings	That rings true
	Sounds	That sounds right

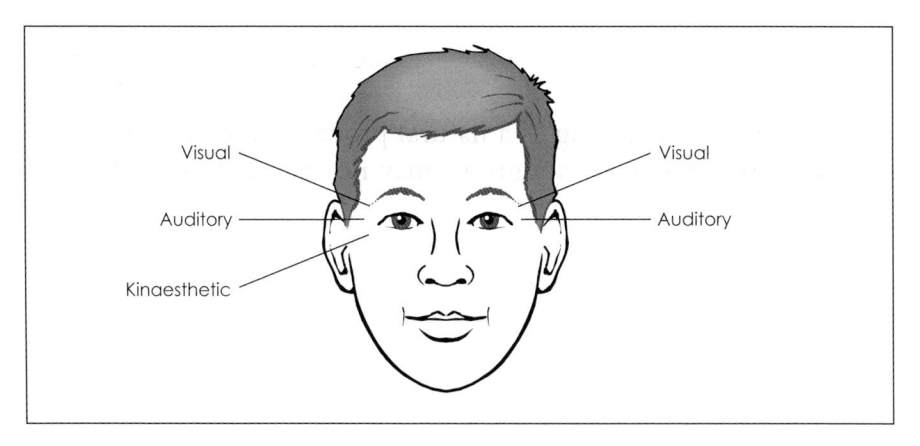

Figure 9.3 Eye movement said to indicate the type of mental process being used by a right handed person

9.3.2 Techniques of NLP

NLP techniques (Bandler et al, 1985; Dilts and De Lozier, 2000) involve pacing non-verbal behaviour (body posture, head position, gestures, voice tone, etc.) and matching speech and body rhythms (breathing, pulse, etc.) and are used to establish and maintain rapport. Strategies include:

i) *Anchoring*: This is a process in which a positive state or response to a personal experience is associated with an 'anchor'. An anchor is most often a gesture, a voice tone or a touch but could be any unique stimulus that can trigger a reaction or emotion. The objective is to link a positive state, such as confidence or relaxation, to something that is repeatable in other situations. Anchoring is a natural process that usually occurs without our awareness. It is similar to classical conditioning in as much as anchors are formed by association with a stimulus and reinforced when the stimulus is repeated. For an anchor to be forged the stimulus has to be specific and intermittent and has to be connected to a prompt, specific and unique reaction. 'Anchoring' is a natural process which affects how we feel even though we may not be aware of it. It is used in theatre and film, by, for example, introducing 'mood' music, to evoke psychological changes in the audience. In NLP, it is used to manage a person's state, for example, to overcome fears.

ii) *Reframing*: This is a process of transforming an individual's perception by giving a positive intention to an undesirable behaviour. A positive alternative is found and used to resolve conflict and implement new behaviour. In psychotherapy, irrational beliefs are often challenged by the therapist on the basis of evidence, leading to reframing experiences in a more realistic way.

An NLP technique, known as the 'six step reframe', is based on the idea that there is a positive intention behind all behaviours. A staged process is used to identify the intention and create alternative choices to satisfy that intention. The six stages are:

1. Identification of the behaviour needing change
2. Communication with the part causing the behaviour
3. Identification of the positive intent behind the behaviour
4. Generation of possible alternative behaviours which will satisfy the intent
5. Choosing three favoured replacement behaviours
6. Checking to see if there is any other internal conflict regarding the change.

A mild hypnotic trance state is used by NLP practitioners during which unconscious resources are drawn upon to effect the change. This is intended to allow an unwanted behaviour or bad habit to be replaced with a more desirable one without losing the benefits of the old behaviour.

iii) *Parts integration*: This involves identifying internal conflicts. In order to resolve these, each aspect is negotiated with separately and then together. Successful parts negotiation involves listening to and negotiating with the different aspects in order to reach a resolution which meets the needs of each.

9.3.3 NLP as a way of thinking

Neurolinguistic programming techniques were originally developed for use in therapy and remain in use in the fields of therapy and of business training. Although NLP claims to be based on cognitive psychology, neurophysiology, linguistics, systems theory and computer science, its association with science is very controversial. NLP is perhaps better viewed as a way of thinking which focuses on helping clients overcome their own subjective problems. Some ideas from NLP may be useful to the audiologist in the counselling process.

Chapter 10
Evaluation

10.1 QUANTIFYING SUCCESS

Rehabilitation of the hearing impaired client most usually involves hearing aids and counselling. Rehabilitation will only be really effective if it addresses the needs that the client perceives. The audiologist must therefore be able to assist the client to identify their problem areas in relation to hearing loss and to establish their goals. When goals have been set, an audiologic plan can be decided with stated specific desired outcomes and the degree of success achieved can then be measured.

Clients' communication difficulties pre-hearing aid fitting can be grouped into the following categories:

1. The quality of the speech signal reaching the client.
2. The client's speech processing ability.
3. The client's speech recognition capability (understanding and knowledge).
4. The client's ability to manage the communication environment.
5. The client's personality and their attitude towards communication repair.

Considering these areas may help in the choice of appropriate evaluation measures. Hearing aid verification procedures, such as real ear measures and functional gain can be used to evaluate the degree to which the technical hearing aid goals have been met. Factor analysis of hearing aid outcomes (Humes, 1999) has suggested that aided speech recognition performance is a major factor in outcome measurement. Subjective satisfaction and benefit ratings are also important.

'In an ideal environment, it could be envisaged that a target for each hearing aid fitting would be for the listener to use their hearing aid all of the time, report hearing as perfect with their hearing aid, no residual difficulty and be delighted with their hearing aid for each of the listening situations relevant to their experience and which, prior to intervention, led to hearing difficulty. However, such a goal is likely to remain unachievable...' (Gatehouse 1997).

Quantifying success should be part of the rehabilitation process, although outcome measures such as self-report questionnaires are not widely used routinely (Lindley, 2006). In order to use outcome measures, information is often obtained pre and post hearing aid fitting, the difference being the degree of success. An evaluation that provides information on difficulties that remain to be addressed will also be useful. The timing of such an evaluation will depend upon the purpose but, if the client is to be acclimatised to hearing aids before evaluation, the evaluation will ideally take place about two to three months after fitting.

10.2 SELF-ASSESSMENT MEASURES OF EVALUATION

10.2.1 Measures available

Self-assessment measures should provide a simple, relatively quick, non-invasive and inexpensive evaluation tool. The measure chosen should be related to the client's specific problem areas and be appropriate to their environment, for example a questionnaire suitable for an active adult might well be unsuitable for a nursing home resident. When using a short evaluation, small differences between scores in the unaided and aided conditions are unlikely to be statistically significant. Nevertheless, self-assessment measures are viewed as a useful addition to the assessment test battery and can provide information about a client's reaction to hearing loss and to hearing aids that cannot be obtained from audiometric measures alone.

Self-assessment measures may be used to indicate:

- Where communication breakdowns exist
- How the significant others feel about these (their views may be quite different from those of the client!)
- How the client feels about their hearing loss
- The degree of hearing aid benefit.

This information can be very helpful in planning the rehabilitation programme. Many measures are available but no single measure addresses every area of need.

Most self-assessment measures are criterion referenced or norm referenced (or both). *Criterion referencing* compares the client's ratings on two separate occasions, which will usually be before and after hearing aid fitting.

Norm referencing compares the client's score to those of a sample of a normative population, for example a representative sample of new hearing aid users.

The measure to be used has to be selected by the audiologist from those available, examples of which are shown in *Table 10.1*. A brief description of some of these follows.

Table 10.1 Examples of self-assessment measures

Abbreviation	Measure Title
COSI	The Client Orientated Scale of Improvement
APHAB	The Abbreviated Profile of Hearing Aid Benefit
GHAPB	The Glasgow Hearing Aid Benefit Profile
GHADP	The Glasgow Hearing Aid Difference Profile
HHIE	The Hearing Handicap Inventory for the Elderly
HHIA	The Hearing Handicap Inventory for Adults
HHS	The Hearing Handicap Scale
DSCF	The Denver Scale of Communication Function
HPI	The Hearing Performance Inventory
SAC	Self Assessment of Communication
SOAC	Significant Other Assessment of Communication
CPI	Communication Profile for the Hearing Impaired

10.2.2 The Abbreviated Profile of Hearing Aid Benefit (APHAB)

The Abbreviated Profile of Hearing Aid Benefit (APHAB), (Cox and Alexander, 1995), is a shortened version of the Profile of Hearing Aid Benefit (Cox and Gilmore, 1990). APHAB consists of 24 items in which clients report the amount of trouble

Evaluation

they are having with communication or noise in various everyday situations. Hearing aid benefit can be calculated by comparing the client's reported difficulty unaided and aided. The profile includes four subscales:

1. Ease of Communication (EC)
2. Reverberation (RV)
3. Background Noise (BN)
4. Aversiveness (AV), i.e. negative reactions to environmental sounds.

Within each subscale there are six sentences to which the client has to answer (A to G) according to the amount of time that the statement is true for them, see *Table 10.2*. The answers that come closest to the client's everyday experience are circled. The following is an example from each subscale. (The specific subscale is given in brackets):

- I have to ask people to repeat themselves in a one-to-one conversation in a quiet room. (EC)
- I have trouble understanding others when an air conditioner or fan is on. (BN)
- I miss a lot of information when I am listening to a lecture. (RV)
- Unexpected sounds, like a smoke detector or alarm bell, are uncomfortable. (AV)

Table 10.2 The choices for each APHAB situation

	A	B	C	D	E	F	G
Amount of time	Always	Almost always	Generally	Almost all the time	Occasionally	Seldom	Never
Percentage (NB Some items reverse the scoring system)	99%	87%	75%	50%	25%	12%	1%

10.2.3 The Glasgow Hearing Aid Benefit Profile (GHABP)

The Glasgow Hearing Aid Benefit Profile (Gatehouse, 1999) is one of few British measures (most are American). It considers disability and benefit and is designed for use in routine clinical practice, both for individual client management and as part of a quality assurance programme. The profile is completed by interview and covers a number of specified listening situations (including up to four that are particularly important to the client), for example:

- Listening to the television with family or friends when the volume is adjusted to suit other people.
- Carrying on a conversation in a busy street.

Only listening situations that exist for the client are included. For each situation there are six questions which relate to:

1. Initial auditory disability, i.e. the degree of difficulty experienced prior to management.
2. Initial auditory handicap, i.e. the impact on the client's life prior to management.

3. Hearing aid use, i.e. the extent to which the hearing aid is used in that listening situation.
4. Hearing aid benefit, i.e. extent to which hearing is improved by the hearing aid in that listening situation.
5. Residual disability, i.e. hearing difficulty remaining in that listening situation after hearing aid fitting.
6. Hearing aid satisfaction, i.e. with their hearing aid in that listening situation.

Each question (e.g. How much difficulty do you have in this situation?) is marked on a 5 point scale, where 1 means 'No difficulty' and 5 means 'Cannot manage at all', see *Table 10.3*. The first two questions (for each situation) are usually completed at the assessment visit, prior to hearing aid fitting, and the remaining four questions are completed at follow up. However the audiologist may choose to complete all the questions at follow up.

Table 10.3 *The choices for a GHABP situation*

Does this situation happen in your life?
0_ No   1_ Yes

How much difficulty do you have in this situation?	How much does any difficulty in this situation worry, annoy or upset you?	In this situation, what proportion of the time do you wear your hearing aid?	In this situation, how much does your hearing aid help you?	In this situation, with your hearing aid, how much difficulty do you now have?	For this situation, how satisfied are you with your hearing aid?
0_ N/A	0_ N/A	0_ N/A	0_ N/A	0_ N/A	0_ N/A
1_ No difficulty	1_ Not at all	1_ Never/not at all	1_ Hearing aid no use at all	1_ No difficulty	1_ Not satisfied at all
2_ Only slightly difficult	2_ Only a little	2_ About ¼ of the time	2_ Hearing aid some help	2_ Only slightly difficult	2_ A little satisfied
3_ Moderate difficulty	3_ A moderate amount	3_ About ½ of the time	3_ Hearing aid is quite helpful	3_ Moderate difficulty	3_ Reasonably satisfied
4_ Great difficulty	4_ Quite a lot	4_ About ¾ of the time	4_ Hearing aid is great help	4_ Great difficulty	4_ Very satisfied
5_ Cannot manage at all	5_ Very much indeed	5_ All the time	5_ Hearing is perfect with aid	5_ Cannot manage at all	5_ Delighted with aid

The Glasgow Hearing Aid Difference Profile (**GHADP**) is an adaptation of the Glasgow Hearing Aid Benefit Profile used for existing hearing aid users when a change in prescription is being implemented and evaluated.

10.2.4 The Hearing Handicap Inventory for the Elderly (HHIE)

The Hearing Handicap Inventory for the Elderly (HHIE), (Ventry and Weinstein, 1982), is a self-assessment questionnaire consisting of 25 items, designed to assess the psychosocial effects of hearing impairment in elderly people. There are two subscales:

- The emotional consequences of hearing impairment; (13 items).
- The social and situational effects of hearing impairment; (12 items).

Scoring is done by awarding 0 to 'no', 2 to 'sometimes' and 4 to 'yes'. The maximum score is 100 and the higher the score obtained the greater is the perceived handicap. A shortened version of ten items, known as the **Hearing Handicap Inventory for the Elderly Screening version** (**HHIE-S**), can be used for screening purposes. A further modification to the original was made for adults under 65 which includes occupational questions.

10.2.5 The Hearing Aid Performance Inventory (HAPI)

The Hearing Aid Performance Inventory (Walden et al, 1984) consists of 64 situational items intended to quantify hearing aid benefit after a period of use (i.e. not pre and post fitting). The items are differentiated into:

- Noisy listening situations
- Quiet situations with listener in close proximity
- Situations with reduced signal information
- Situations with non-speech stimuli.

After hearing aid fitting the client is asked to rate the help given by the hearing aid in particular communication environments, for example:

'You are involved in an intimate conversation with your spouse.'

Responses can range on a five point scale to indicate that in this situation, the hearing aid is from 'very helpful' (1) to it 'hinders performance'(5). Scoring involves adding all the numbers together, dividing by the number of items and multiplying by 20 to give a percentage. A low score indicates a good performance. The normative group data is based on 119 men and 9 women who had sloping sensorineural losses and wore their aids on average 10.8 hours per day.

A shortened version (**SHAPI**) consisting of 38 situations is also available.

10.2.6 The Client Orientated Scale of Improvement (COSI)

The Client Orientated Scale of Improvement was produced by Dillon, James and Ginis (1997). Scores are compared with the degree of benefit expected in a comparable population in a similar situation. The normative population used was 1,770 hearing impaired adults including over 50% who were new hearing aid users. It utilises sixteen standardised situations of which five are chosen by the client in discussion with the audiologist. The situations identify where the client would particularly like to manage better and must be very specific, for example:

'I want to hear better when listening to the teacher at evening class'.

Each situation is ranked in order of importance and at the follow up appointment the client has to judge the degree of change for each situation due to the hearing aids, for example:

'Because of the new hearing aids I now hear... (worse, no difference, slightly better, better, much better)'.

They also have to note their final ability with the aids by completing:

'I can hear satisfactorily ... (hardly ever, occasionally, half the time, most of the time, almost always)'

If COSI is used during the planning stage of rehabilitation, it can assist the audiologist to identify goals for the rehabilitation programme.

10.2.7 The Hearing Performance Inventory (HPI)

The Hearing Performance Inventory (HPI), (Giolas, Owens, Lamb and Schubert, 1979), was developed to assess hearing performance in a number of everyday listening situations covering a variety of speaker characteristics and communication processes. The questionnaire has six sections:

- Understanding Speech
- Intensity
- Response to Auditory Failure

- Social
- Personal
- Occupational.

It is administered in an interview format, which is estimated to take about 35 minutes. To score, the numbers are added and divided by the number of items answered and multiplied by 20, to give a percentage. The best score is 0% (no difficulty) and 100% indicates the most difficulty.

The advantage of the HPI is that it was rigorously developed but unfortunately its length tends to make it impractical. The scores from individual areas, particularly from the Understanding Speech and Intensity sections, may be more useful than the global scores (Lamb et al, 1983).

There is also a revised version (**HPI-R**) in which the number of items is reduced to 90. This can be further reduced if the client is not employed by omitting the occupational area (Johnson and Danhauer, 2002). Administration of the revised version without the occupational section takes about 20 minutes.

Chapter 11
Assistive Devices

11.1 THE NEED FOR ASSISTIVE DEVICES

Although digital hearing aids are technologically advanced instruments, designed to counteract the effects of noise to a great extent, they do not fully correct hearing. Hearing aids perform best when the person speaking is close by and there is little interfering noise. Some situations in which hearing aids cannot overcome the communication problems sufficiently well will usually still remain, and in these other devices to supplement or replace conventional hearing aids may greatly assist. Difficult listening situations generally involve background noise, distance from the sound source and reverberation. However, the precise situations where assistive devices can help will depend on the individual's hearing loss, lifestyle and needs.

Background noise interferes with hearing the required speech signal or other sound. Noise interferes with everyone's ability to hear well but is particularly destructive for people with hearing impairments. In order to hear satisfactorily hearing impaired listeners require a better signal-to-noise ratio (a quieter situation) than their normally hearing counterparts. In general their signal-to-noise ratio needs to be about 15dB better than that required with normal hearing.

Distance from the sound source causes difficulty for hearing impaired listeners because the further away the listener is from the sound source, the quieter the sound will be and, in addition, the less easy it will be to lipread. Sound loses intensity (volume) rapidly as it travels away from the source, so that even a relatively short distance away can cause difficulty for the hearing impaired listener, particularly in situations of background noise, see *Figure 11.1*.

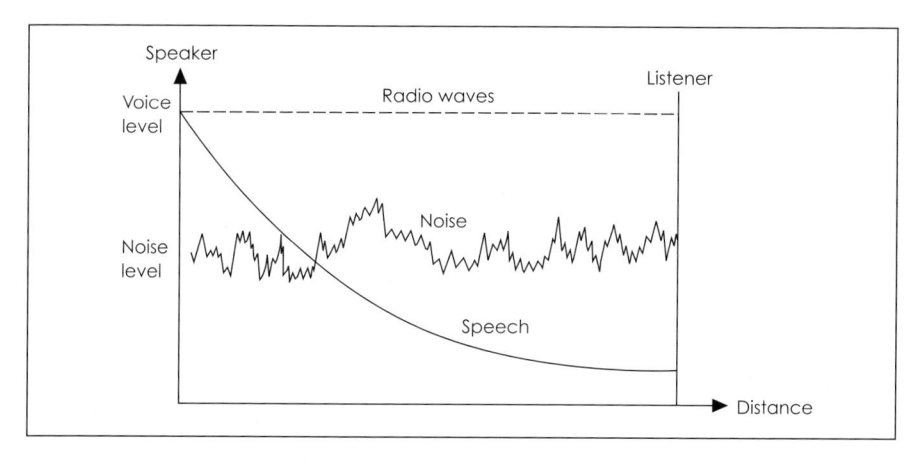

Figure 11.1 *Loss of sound intensity with distance (Reproduced with kind permission of Maltby 2002)*

Reverberation is the continuance of sound due to reflections. Swimming pools, churches, gymnasia or large halls are reverberant places. Hard surfaces reflect sound and degrade the signal. This is not a great problem with normal hearing unless the reverberation time (that is the time taken for the noise to die away) is very long. For hearing aid users the effect of reverberation on listening is much worse as the direct signal and the reflected signal may arrive at the microphone at different times, making speech difficult to understand.

Some situations are so difficult that the hearing impaired person may try to avoid them altogether. However there are many devices available to assist. These can be grouped into:

1. Alerting devices
2. Assistive listening devices (including devices for television, radio and other one-way listening devices and for telephone use)
3. Alternative communication devices.

11.2 TYPES OF ASSISTIVE DEVICES

11.2.1 Alerting devices

These are warning devices. They may use amplified sound or an alternative frequency (such as a low frequency buzzer for someone with a high frequency hearing loss) or some other method of conveying the signal, such as vibration or flashing lights. There are devices available, see *Figure 11.2*, for the telephone, alarm clocks, smoke alarms, burglar alarms, doorbells, etc. The device can be placed where it is most helpful, for example a flashing device to warn of the doorbell or telephone could be placed in the kitchen and/or the lounge.

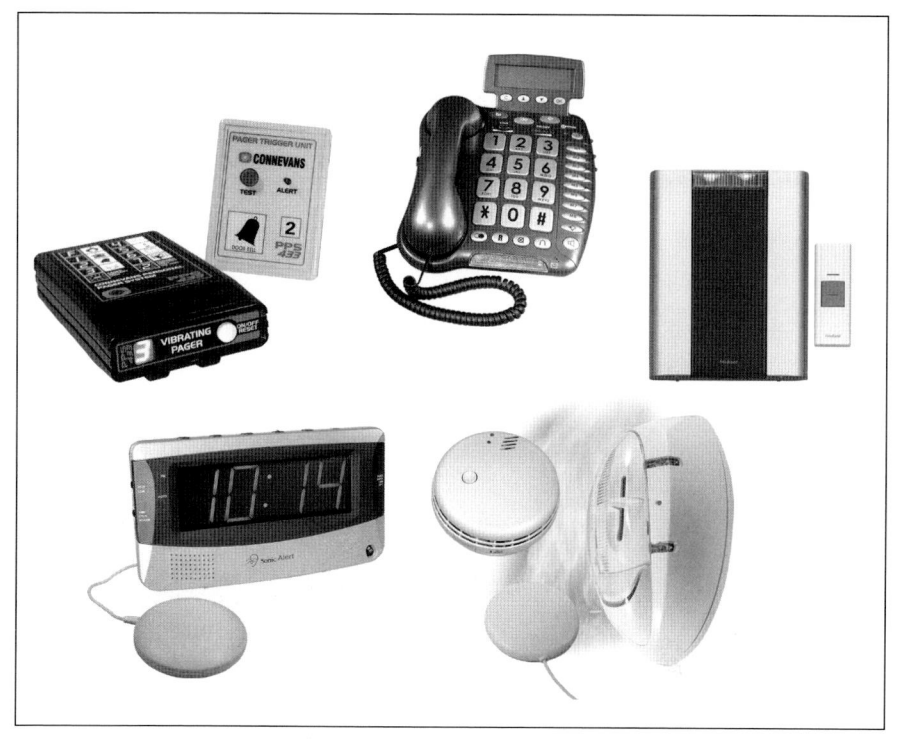

Figure 11.2 *A selection of alerting devices (Kindly supplied by Connevans Ltd)*

11.2.2 Assistive listening devices

Assistive listening devices (ALDs) are designed to overcome the effects of distance, background noise and reverberation. There are many different assistive devices available to satisfy the wide range of difficult listening situations that exist for people. Those people who find them useful may use them in addition to, or instead of, hearing aids. Devices may be hardwired (attached physically) or connected wirelessly.

Hearing aids may be linked to assistive listening devices wirelessly by telecoil or a radio link. A radio link may be made

Assistive Devices 199

via direct audio input (DAI). Direct audio input can also be linked to a device by a plug or via an audio shoe and a plug, see *Figure 11.3*. The audio shoe and plug, see *Figure 11.4*, are not all standardised and must be of the appropriate type to match the particular hearing aid.

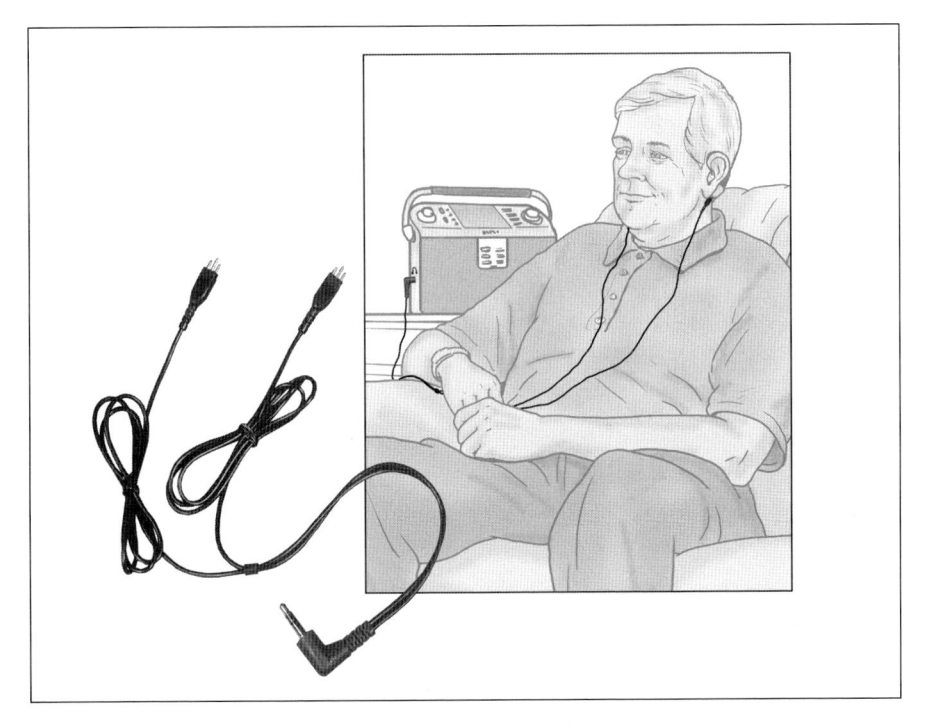

Figure 11.3 *Direct audio input (Kindly supplied by Connevans Ltd)*

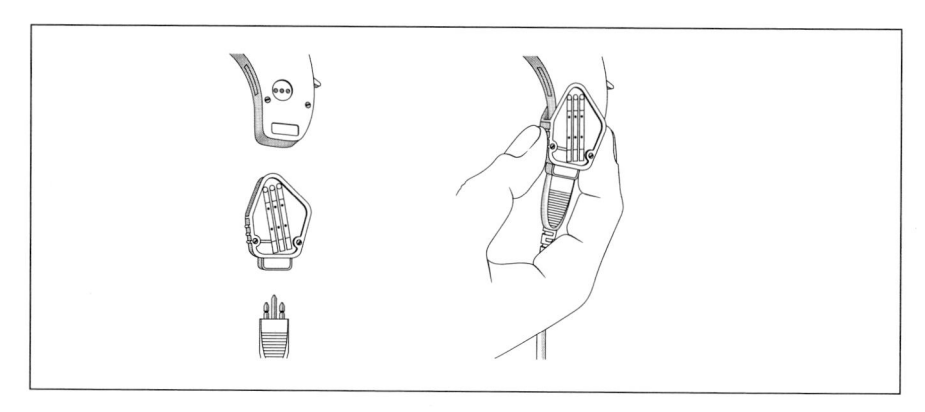

Figure 11.4 A shoe and plug being attached to a post aural hearing aid

i) Listening to television and radio

The television is commonly used by hearing impaired people at a volume which is too loud for others in the vicinity. This can be overcome by using a portable amplifier and neck loop, see *Figure 11.5*, or a wireless system. The latter has the advantage of not involving trailing wires which could present a safety hazard.

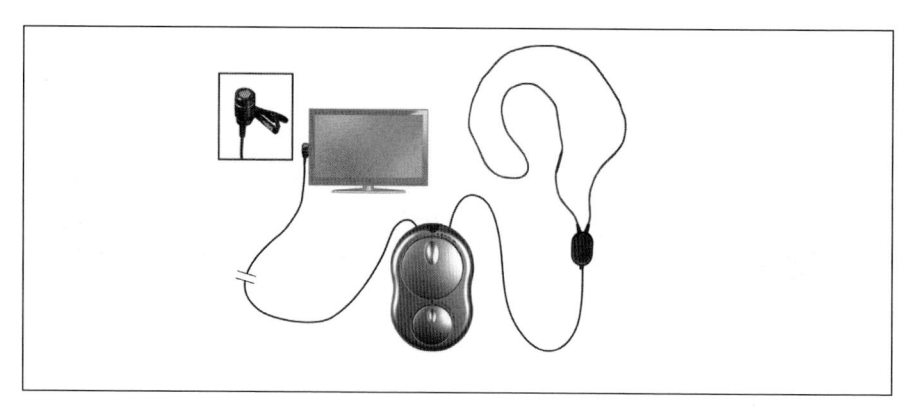

Figure 11.5 A portable amplifier and neck loop for the television (Kindly supplied by Connevans Ltd)

ii) Telephone use

Some hearing impaired people use amplifying devices; others use devices that communicate through text. Amplified telephones are available with volume controls. Telephones are also available, see *Figure 11.6*, with an inductive loop facility, or a portable inductive loop coupler may be used, although these are less efficient. Some hearing aids can be connected by bluetooth to provide a hands free system. Use of a webcam in conjunction with phone conversations made via the internet can provide lipread cues. Special text phones can be used to facilitate typed conversations, which appear as a readout display or which may be printed. The Royal National Institute for the Deaf (RNID) manages a 'Type Talk' service for deaf people (or others with communication difficulties), which is a national telephone relay service. It allows a hearing person to speak their part of a conversation whilst an operator types what is being said and relays it to the text phone, see *Figure 11.7*, of the deaf participant. The deaf person can reply directly, by speaking to the hearing person, or type their reply for the operator to read out. Normal mobile phones, whilst not specifically for deaf people, can of course also be used for simple text messaging.

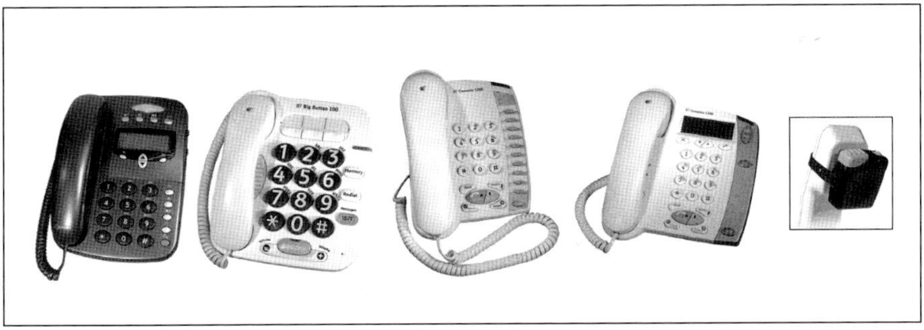

Figure 11.6 *Telephones may have an inductive loop facility (Kindly supplied by Connevans Ltd)*

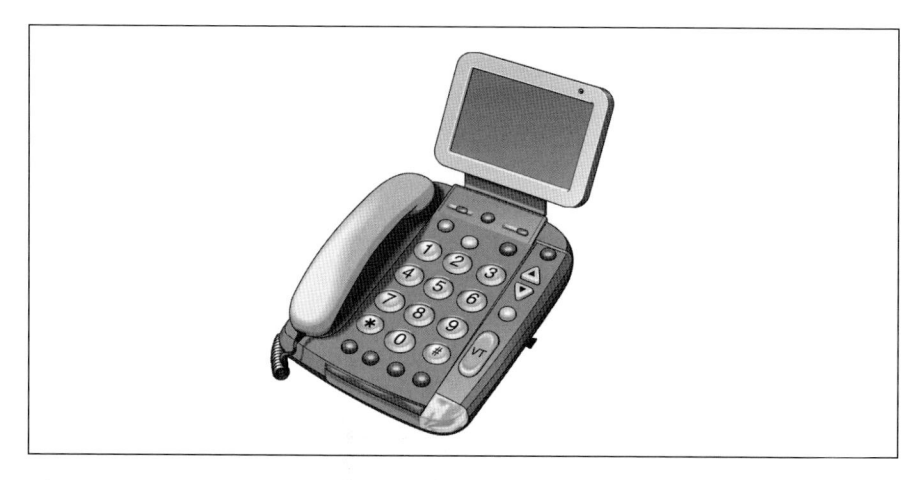

Figure 11.7 *A text phone (Kindly supplied by Connevans Ltd)*

11.2.3. Alternative communication devices

These are mainly designed for profoundly deaf people who gain little help from hearing aids, see *Figure 11.8*. These individuals particularly may benefit from assistive devices based on tactile or visual stimuli. However there are times when people with less severe hearing losses will also benefit from alternative communication devices, for example when needing to be aware of a particular sound from another place, or despite a noisy environment, or to be awakened from sleep. They are useful for being alerted to doorbells, baby alarms, telephones, fire alarms, alarm clocks, timers, etc. The systems may be permanently positioned or placed temporarily, for example under the pillow at night. The system may monitor one or many signals and may also be linked to a wireless vibrating pager that can be carried on the person. Whilst not really a 'device', trained hearing dogs are also used by some deaf people to alert them to the various sounds in the environment.

Assistive Devices 203

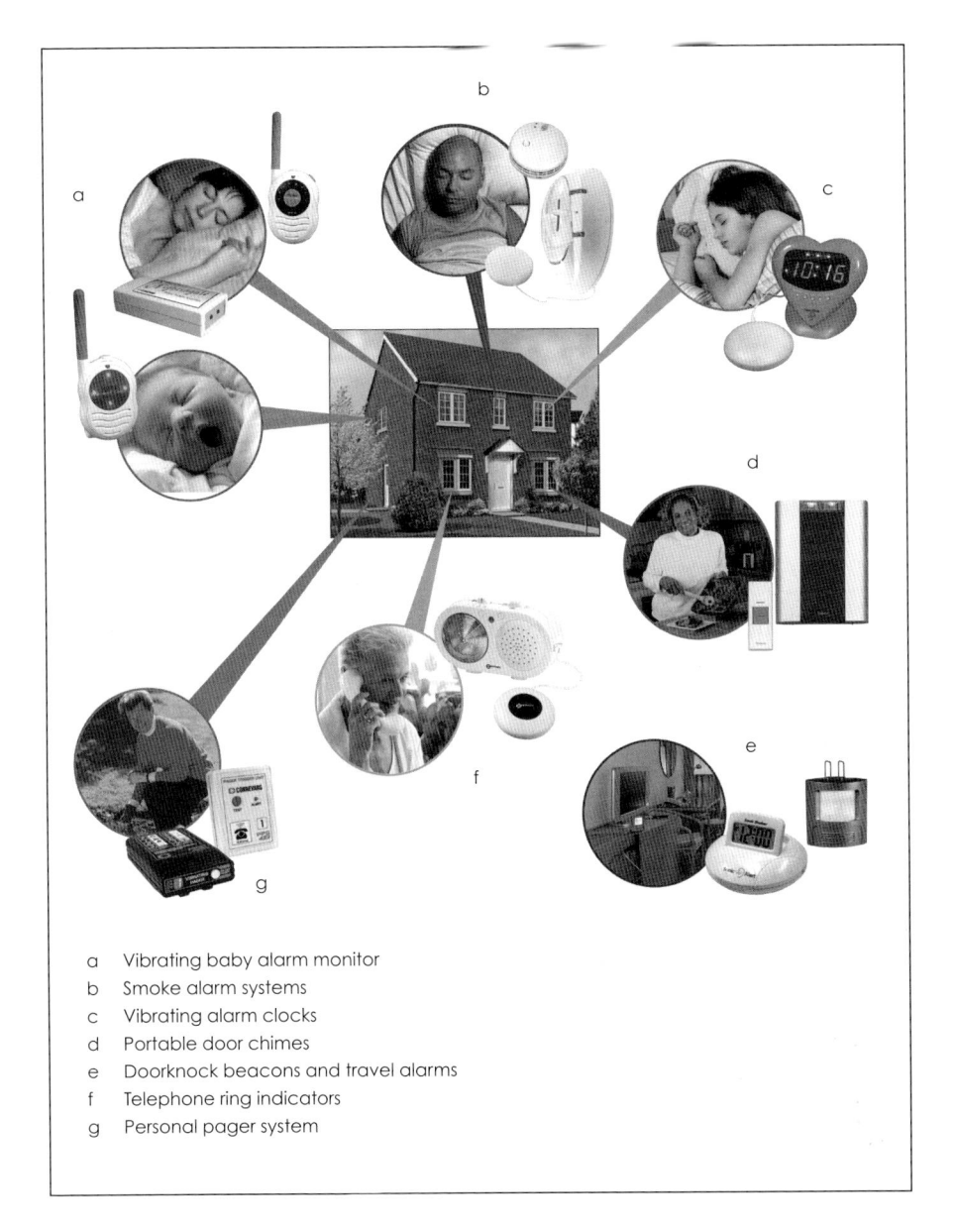

a Vibrating baby alarm monitor
b Smoke alarm systems
c Vibrating alarm clocks
d Portable door chimes
e Doorknock beacons and travel alarms
f Telephone ring indicators
g Personal pager system

Figure 11.8 Examples of alternative communication devices (Kindly supplied by Connevans Ltd)

The simplest device for one-to-one conversation is a pencil and paper, with each person making notes that are passed between them. In meetings or lectures it is helpful to obtain notes in advance, as awareness of the subject matter will make it easier to follow the lecture or discussion. If someone can point to where the speaker is up to, this will keep the deaf person on track. Subtitles or captions are available for many films and television programmes in place of (or in addition to) hearing. Some television programmes are available with a signed version given in the corner.

11.3 WIRELESS SYSTEMS

A wireless system provides sound direct to the hearing aid, thus overcoming the problems of distance from the sound source, reverberation and background noise. However from the auditory signal alone, the user cannot tell which direction the sound is coming from. In some situations the use of some form of visual signalling, or spoken identification by name, may help the user to identify who is speaking.

11.3.1 The induction loop system

In the loop system, see *Figure 11.9*, the sound signal from a microphone is converted to an electrical signal, amplified and fed through a loop of wire. This causes an electromagnetic field within the loop. The magnetic signals within the loop are an analogue of the sound signals, that is they vary in strength and frequency exactly as the sound signal. A hearing aid fitted with a telecoil will pick up the magnetic signals when set to the 'T' position. The magnetic signals are then converted back to sound signals and delivered to the ear. Anyone within the loop with an active telecoil should receive a good signal. Someone without an active telecoil will receive nothing from the loop and cannot

Assistive Devices

even tell if it is on or off. Telecoil receivers are available in various forms.

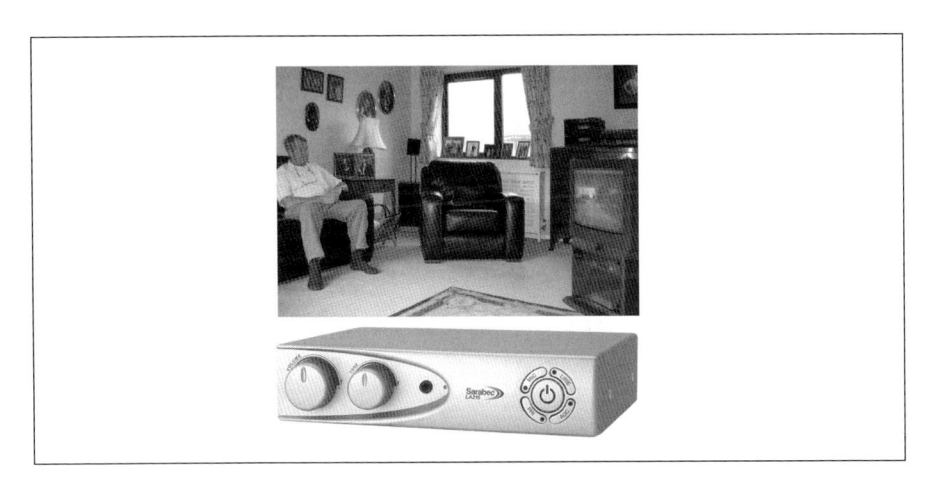

Figure 11.9 A loop system (Kindly supplied by Connevans Ltd)

When using a hearing aid with a loop or 'T' setting, the microphone ('M' setting, see *Figure 11.10*) of the aid is switched off when using the 'T' setting, so that background noise is excluded. Alternatively, with some hearing aids, it can be left active (using an 'MT' setting) so that surrounding sounds can still be heard. Where the hearing aid has been programmed to provide an 'MT' setting, the microphone will usually be set to deliver the surrounding sound at a lower level than the signal received from the loop or 'T'.

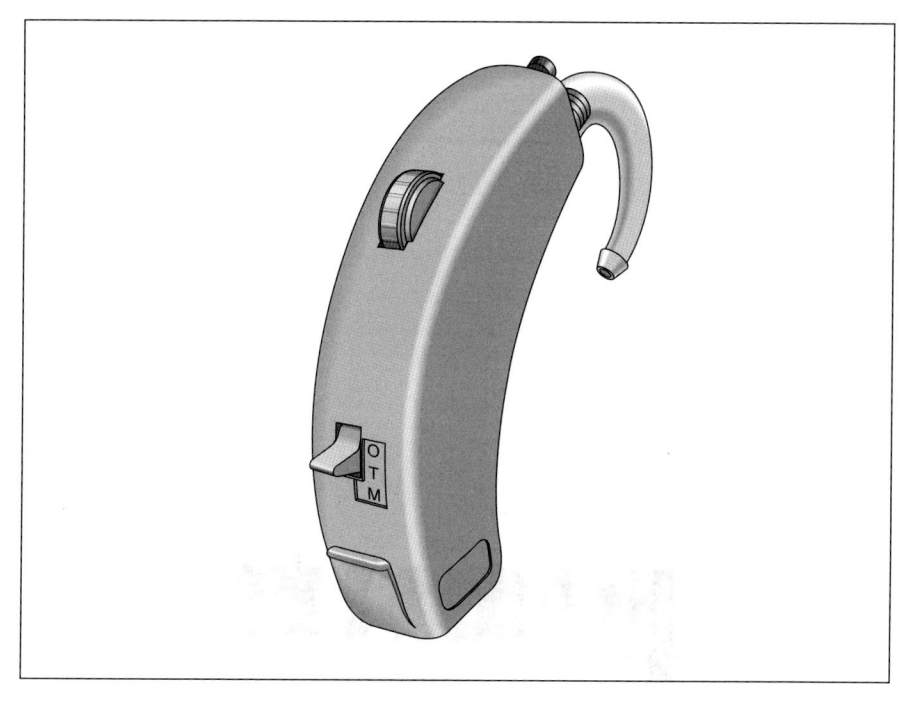

Figure 11.10 *The M and T settings on a hearing aid*

The loop system is relatively inexpensive and maintenance is low. Many people have aids fitted with telecoil and are therefore able to benefit from loop equipment fitted in public places. However, the loop also suffers from a number of possible disadvantages including:

- Interference from electrical hum (from fluorescent lights, transformers and mains wiring).
- Overspill of electromagnetic signals into adjacent areas where it could interfere with another loop system if such was installed.
- Reduced signal with alterations in the telecoil plane, for example by moving the head to one side.

- The low frequency response when using the loop may be less good than with the hearing aid alone. This is only likely to be important with profound hearing losses where the low frequencies are vital to speech reception.
- The loop system may be badly or incorrectly installed and therefore provide a disappointing response for the hearing aid wearer. A loop should comply with the British Standards Code of Practice and should also be regularly checked to ensure that it is working properly and that the field strength is correct.

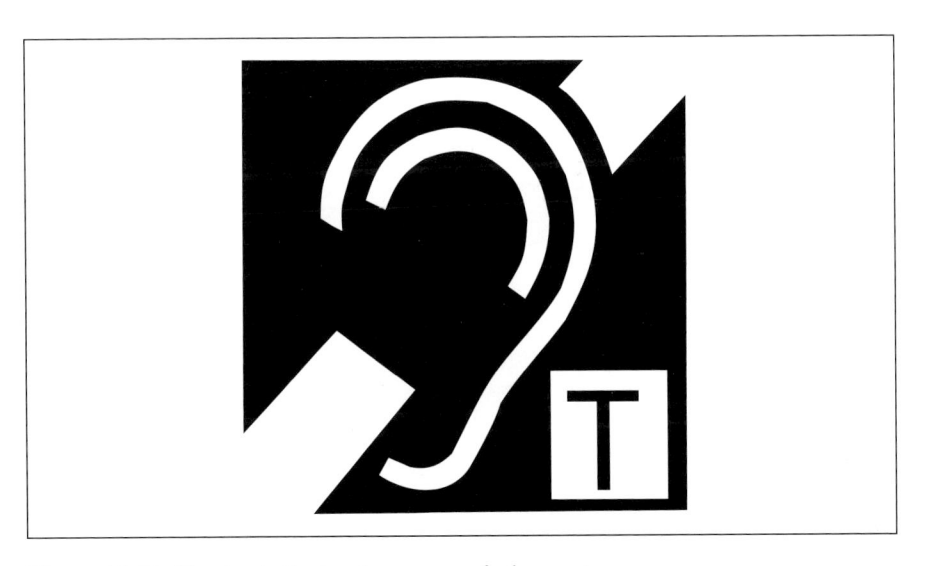

Figure 11.11 The sign indicating the presence of a loop system

Loops can be obtained for the home or for public settings. The home type is typically used for the television. The system consists of a thin wire laid around the room and connected to a small amplifier mounted near the television or linked to it via a jack plug. Many banks, cinemas, railway booking offices and shops have a loop fitted at one or more of their counters. The hearing aid wearer knows to adjust their hearing aid to receive the loop signal when they see the sign shown in *Figure 11.11*. Loops are also commonly placed in theatres, cinemas and churches. Portable loop systems are often used at conferences and for other public meetings. If the whole room is not looped, the listener must be careful to stay within the loop to be sure of obtaining a good signal. Individual wearable loops systems, such as neck loops, see *Figure 11.12*, are also available. This type of loop can be worn under clothes if required to conceal from view.

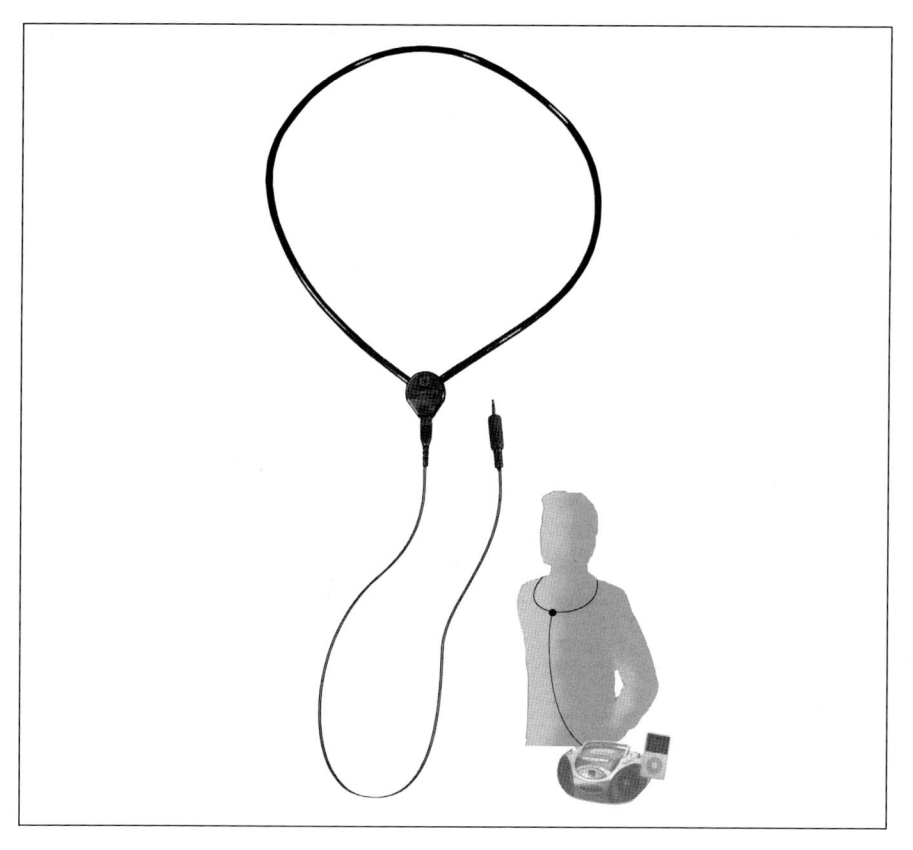

Figure 11.12 *A neck loop (Kindly supplied by Connevans Ltd)*

11.3.2 Infra red systems

An infrared system, see *Figure 11.13*, consists of two parts, a mains powered transmitter and a receiver powered by a rechargeable battery. The transmitter converts the sound signals it receives into infrared (invisible light) signals and transmits them across the room. These signals can be picked up by a photo detector diode (or 'eye') in an infrared receiver worn by the listener. Light travels in straight lines, so must receive direct or reflected light from the transmitter to work, this means that the receiver has to be within the same room as the transmitter. Bright sunlight will interfere with infrared only if it is shining directly on the receptor and so the system can work inside or out although outdoors the transmitter must be in line of sight since there are no suitable surfaces to reflect the signal.

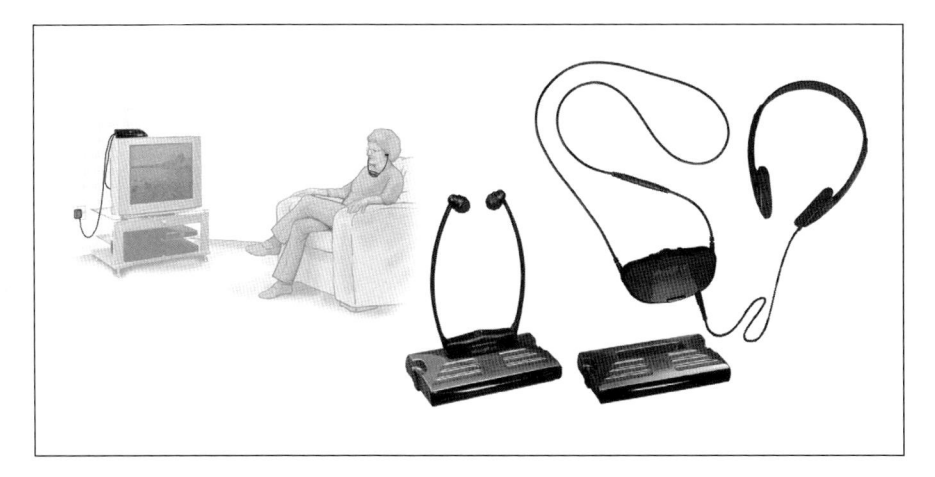

Figure 11.13 *An infrared system (Kindly supplied by Connevans Ltd)*

11.3.3 Frequency modulated (FM) radio aids

All radio aids include a transmitter which receives the sound and converts it to a radio signal. A microphone is an integral part to the transmitter. Most radio aid microphone/transmitters are designed to be worn by someone speaking (usually a teacher or parent). However, some are hand-held or can be placed on a table and can be pointed towards a speaker or passed around a group.

The client wears a receiver that picks up the radio signal and changes it into sound. Most receivers include a volume control, which may be set by the audiologist. Receivers are usually small units that are attached by direct audio input to some hearing aids or cochlear implant processors. Radio aids are widely used by hearing impaired school children.

Radio aids are very versatile, they can be used inside or outside, their signal travels a considerable distance and the use of different frequencies overcomes overspill interference problems. Occasionally radio aids suffer from interference from other radio transmissions; also the equipment is relatively expensive both to buy and to maintain.

Some hearing aids have 'direct audio input', which allows the radio signal to be fed directly into the hearing aid. This produces consistent high-quality sound. If the hearing aids have a 'T' setting but no facility for direct audio input, the receiver can be used with a neck loop, see *Figure 11.14*. The hearing aid is switched to the telecoil ('T' or 'MT') position and the sound from the radio aid can be heard via the loop. Radio aid receivers may be body worn, see *Figure 11.14(a)* or miniaturised in or attached to the hearing aid 'shoe', as in *Figure 11.14(c)*.

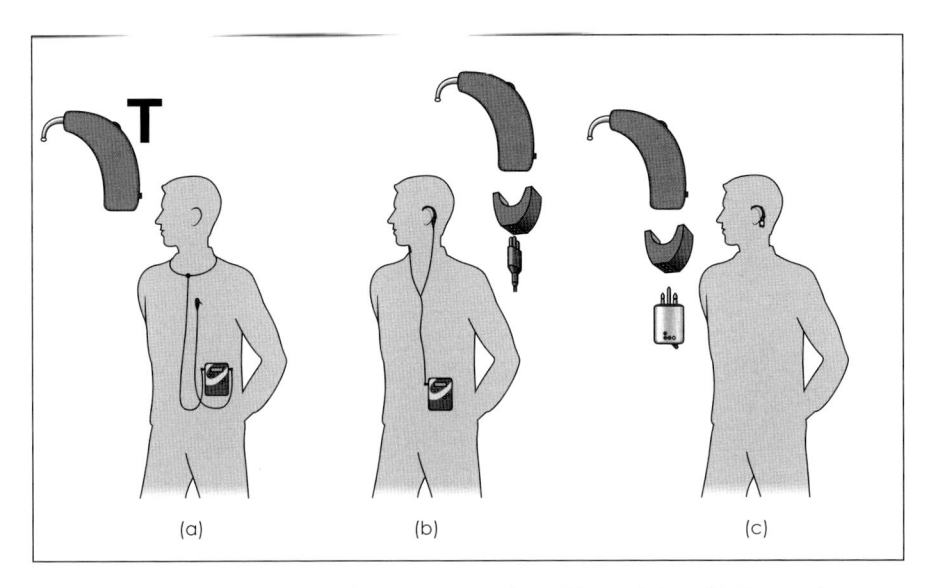

Figure 11.14 *A radio hearing aid system connected via (a) a neck loop (b) direct audio input to body worn receivers (c) ear-worn radio aids*

11.3.4 Assessments for assistive devices

Assessment for assistive devices should be part of the rehabilitation process. The audiologist must therefore be aware of the devices available and be able to match these to the client's lifestyle and needs. Assistive devices are not always required but an analysis of the client's communication needs at home and at work should be carried out in order to make an informed decision. Appropriate assistive devices should be demonstrated and the client should be trained to use any that are chosen. This should also be linked in with counselling and assertiveness training. Assertiveness is often required in order for these devices to be used in the situations where they are most needed. After assistive devices have been provided an evaluation should be carried out to establish the usefulness of the device(s) to the client, with further rehabilitation following where necessary.

Assistive devices may be supplied in some cases by social services. However, where the client purchases them they will usually be eligible to be excluded from paying value added tax (VAT).

11.4 SUPPORT SERVICES

Support services may be available through:

- Social services. All social services have eligibility criteria and a charter that explains the help they can provide and to whom. Social services will assess need and may assist with the provision of assistive devices (on loan), in addition to helping with other needs such as housing and general support. The local authority maintains a register of deaf people but this is voluntary. Registration (or non-registration) does not affect a person's right to services. Social work is usually generic but there are also a small number of social workers who work mainly with deaf adults whose first language is sign. These social workers have additional training in deaf issues and communication skills including British Sign Language (BSL).
- The National Health Service (NHS) deals with the medical management of hearing loss, the provision of hearing aids and rehabilitation. Psychological and psychiatric needs are also usually channelled through the NHS.
- Education services may provide support to children and students. Services that may be available include the provision of specialist equipment, classroom assistants, note takers, interpreters and specialist teaching services. Teachers of the deaf have an additional qualification and expertise in teaching deaf children. They may work with:

1. Hearing impaired pupils on an individual basis
2. Small groups of hearing impaired pupils
3. Mainstream teachers and lecturers in further education
4. Teachers in special schools
5. Parents of young deaf children.

- The preschool, school and college education of hearing impaired children is the responsibility of the local authority. Separate support is available for higher education.
- Financial help may be available for disabled students, for example, through grants and other allowances to help meet the extra course costs, for example a note-taker or specialist equipment. Most universities and colleges have a Disability Advisor who will advise on sources of funding. Applications for the *Disabled Students' Allowance* should be made to the student's Local Education Authority.
- Employment services. Disability Employment Advisors can support hearing impaired individuals in the workplace through the *Access to Work* scheme. They may provide specialist equipment and access to training. They may also liaise with employers to alert them to the needs of their deaf employees and how these needs can be met.
- Voluntary organisations. There are many different voluntary organisations, for example for deaf children, hard of hearing adults, deaf adults, deaf-blind people, people with tinnitus, etc. Their role is normally both political campaigning and individual support. It is important that clients are made aware of the support that can be available from the relevant voluntary organisations, so that they can access these if they so wish. They can provide an opportunity to meet and talk to others with similar problems.

Chapter 12
Tinnitus

12.1 WHAT IS TINNITUS?

Tinnitus is noises in the ear, ears or head with no external cause. On very rare occasions *somatosounds* (body sounds), thought to be due to muscle spasm or to vascular changes, may be audible to others.

The word 'tinnitus' is Latin meaning 'a ringing'. The word was first used by Pliny the Elder (AD 23 - AD 79) in the phrase 'tinnitus aurium' referring to noises in the head! In 1693 'tinnitus aurium' appears as a technical phrase in Blanchard's Physician Dictionary but its first use as an English word on its own is on page 649 of St George's Hospital Report 9 in 1879.

Tinnitus is subjective, that is only heard by the sufferer. The noise heard is usually high frequency but can be low frequency. Descriptions of the tinnitus sound are very varied and include:

- High pitched whistling
- Singing
- Escaping steam
- Single or multiple sounds, e.g. musical notes
- Low pitched noise of the sea
- Rumbling or roaring machinery noise
- Clicking
- Throbbing.

It is normal to experience tinnitus when in a very quiet place but about 5% of the population have troublesome tinnitus. When tinnitus is unilateral it is more common in the left ear than the right. The reason is not known.

12.2 LIVING WITH TINNITUS

Tinnitus, like many other conditions, can be mild, troublesome or severe. Severe tinnitus is extremely distressing.

My whole brain, my whole life in fact, was condensed into one great shrieking whistle that shut off at source all power of thought, all desire for communication, all interest in the outside world, all confidence, all humour, and every shred of capacity for pleasure. I was trapped – imprisoned inside a tight dense claustrophobic bubble of ear-splitting sound... At this stage life grew very black indeed. Before long, and without knowing the complexities of inner ear structure, I wondered quite seriously if I could persuade any surgeon to destroy my hearing altogether. To be stone deaf would be infinitely preferable to this fiendish bombardment. (Hawkridge, 1987)

Tinnitus is worse when the world outside is quiet, when the noises are not drowned or lessened by external sound. Yet, at the same time, loud sounds may be intolerable (due to *loudness recruitment*, that is an abnormally rapid rate of loudness growth). Hyperacusis, an inability to tolerate everyday levels of sound, is present in 40% of people with troublesome tinnitus. Sleep is very difficult because the quiet magnifies the awareness of the internal sounds. Stress increases the tinnitus problem. Tiredness and worry that there may be something radically wrong (e.g. a tumour) only serve to increase stress further.

Chronic (long-lasting) severe tinnitus is 'a frequent condition, which can have enormous impact on a patient's life

Tinnitus

and which is very difficult to treat' (Landgrebe et al, 2008). Tinnitus may cause irritation, bad temper, tiredness, anxiety, lack of concentration and other psychological problems. Depression and tinnitus are, not surprisingly, commonly linked. Tolerance of tinnitus noise varies widely. Personality factors impact on the perceived severity of tinnitus (Langguth et al, 2007) but most people tend to become more tolerant of it over time – as they habituate to it. The noise is still there and the level has not changed but the individual begins to ignore it or notice it less. Tinnitus commonly occurs with hearing loss. Many people who are deaf from birth have always suffered from it but in most cases they consider it as normal and do not even realise that tinnitus is not experienced by everyone. However, some congenitally deaf children do complain of noises and find them upsetting. In general, individuals with lesser hearing losses are most likely to be aware of tinnitus.

12.3 HYPERSENSITIVITY

With normal hearing, a person can hear very quiet sounds (about 0dBHL) and tolerate very loud sounds (about 90-115dBHL) without discomfort. With a hearing loss the individual cannot hear quiet sounds and may be less able to tolerate loud sounds due to recruitment, which is very common with sensorineural hearing loss due to cochlear damage.

Even with normal or near normal hearing, some people with tinnitus also suffer from *hyperacusis*, which is discomfort from noises that are not usually at all troublesome with normal hearing. People with hyperacusis also often have misophonia and may develop phonophobia. *Misophonia* is a dislike of normal environmental sounds, whilst *phonophobia* is a fear of normal environmental sounds, such as loud speech, traffic or even doors closing. Social life can be severely disrupted by these conditions as many normal environments may be intolerable.

12.4 TINNITUS PATHOLOGY

12.4.1 Causes of tinnitus

Tinnitus takes a variety of forms and can be due to a number of different causes. Research now suggests that auditory and non-auditory brain areas are involved in tinnitus pathology (Kleinjung et al, 2008). Many disorders that involve the auditory system directly or indirectly can lead to the emergence of tinnitus but, for many clients, the cause of their tinnitus remains unknown. Where it is possible, the site of the problem should be found so that any appropriate medical or surgical treatment can follow. In most cases, investigations only exclude certain causes rather than finding the actual site.

Troublesome or severe tinnitus is often associated with changes in the central auditory system. The normal mechanism of hearing is that the brain interprets changing neuronal signals from the cochlea as sound. These changing signals are usually the result of external sounds. The pitch or frequency of a sound is perceived from the precise location of the inner hair cells that send the signal, see *Figure 12.1*. In the normal auditory system, the place of the neuronal signal from the cochlea is maintained throughout the auditory pathway (this is known as 'tonotopic' organisation). When hair cells in a particular region are destroyed, neuronal activity from that region ceases, 'silent neurons' are present throughout the auditory pathway and the corresponding area in the cortex of the brain does not respond to sound. However after some time (several months) the tonotopic arrangement is altered and the neurons are no longer silent but have tuned into regions around the edge of the hearing loss. These changes in brain activity, with over-representation of those frequencies around the edge of the loss, may lead to spontaneous neural activity or 'hyperexcitability syndrome' (Eichhammer, 2007). This can give rise to tinnitus of a frequency close to that of the person's greatest hearing loss. The sensation of tinnitus may be an auditory phantom perception (Bartels et al, 2007). This is similar to phantom limb sensation (pain, itching, etc. in the non-existent limb), which some people experience after losing a limb.

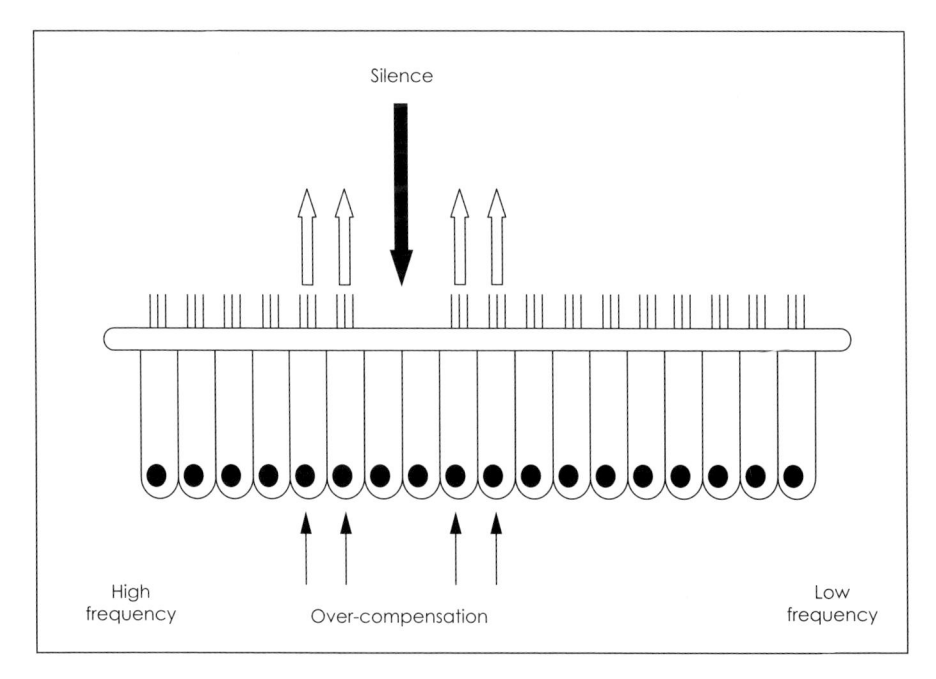

Figure 12.1 Place theory

Tinnitus may occur spontaneously but if the change in background neural activity is sufficiently slow, the brain can adapt to the new pattern, unless or until some other factor upsets the adaptation process and triggers the onset of tinnitus. Triggers may be some form of trauma directly affecting the ear, or they may be something quite trivial such as a perfectly normal ear syringing, or something not obviously related to the ear such as an emotional upset. Some possible causes of tinnitus (or pre-disposing factors) include: impacted wax, ear syringing, high blood pressure, abnormal jaw movement, hearing loss due to cochlear damage, otosclerosis, labyrinthitis, Ménière's syndrome, ototoxicity (drugs that are poisonous to the ear), excessive noise, head injury, nerve damage and tumours.

The human brain is plastic, that is neural activity can change. Research has shown, for example, that:

- Neurons that respond robustly to 4kHz but only weakly to 2kHz can be conditioned to respond maximally to 2kHz (Salvi et al, 2000).
- Colour stimulation can significantly influence auditory perception, red light enhancing loudness perception and green light reducing loudness perception (Hajak et al, 2008).

The brain's neural plasticity may be able to be used successfully in clinical intervention strategies to train the brain to ignore the phantom sounds that are tinnitus.

12.4.2 Medical referral

Tinnitus is usually extremely difficult to describe accurately and measurement of tinnitus is very difficult because of its subjective nature. If tinnitus is severe or troublesome, referral must be made so that a medical examination can be carried out in case the cause of the tinnitus can be medically or surgically treated. Treatments for severe tinnitus are very varied.

12.5 TINNITUS ASSESSMENT

A tinnitus handicap assessment will include a very thorough case history including:

- The onset and duration of the tinnitus.
- A description of the tinnitus.
- The effect on the individual's life (which may include completion of a tinnitus handicap questionnaire, see *Table 12.1*).
- The client's expectations regarding tinnitus treatment/therapy.
- Any history of otalgia (ear pain), noise exposure, head trauma, diabetes, migraine, stroke, high blood pressure, neck problems, etc.
- Any history of family members having troublesome tinnitus.
- Any medications being taken.
- Details of any known hearing loss or other ear problems.
- Any history of dizziness.

Table 12.1 *Some examples of questions from the Tinnitus Handicap Inventory (Newman et al, 1996)*

	Yes	No	Sometimes
Because of your tinnitus, is it difficult for you to concentrate?			
Does the loudness of your tinnitus make it difficult for you to hear people?			
Does your tinnitus make you angry?			
Does your tinnitus make you confused?			
Because of your tinnitus, do you feel desperate?			
Do you complain a great deal about your tinnitus?			
Because of your tinnitus, do you have trouble falling asleep at night?			

An audiometric assessment will usually also be carried out, including for example otoscopic examination, pure tone audiometry and tympanometry. Testing of the tinnitus itself is limited but may involve tinnitus matching, to determine the approximate pitch and loudness of the tinnitus, and applying masking noise to find the minimum level that will block (fully or partially) the tinnitus sound. Tinnitus is almost always less than 20dBSL (sensation level) above the person's hearing threshold level and therefore very high levels of masking should not be necessary and should not be used.

Measuring aspects of tinnitus such as the pitch and loudness can be very beneficial:

- To confirm to the client that their tinnitus is real
- To help in the fitting of hearing aids and/or maskers
- To monitor changes in the tinnitus over time
- To determine reliability in legal cases.

12.6 CURRENT TINNITUS MANAGEMENT STRATEGIES

12.6.1 Medical and surgical treatments

Figure 12.2 shows a possible route for tinnitus sufferers. Medications, e.g. antidepressants, may be used to treat the symptoms of tinnitus. Certain drugs may act as inhibitors to tinnitus but generally the drugs currently available treat the symptoms rather than reducing the tinnitus itself. In some instances, surgical treatment, e.g. destruction of the labyrinth, nerve section and cochlear implantation provides relief but there are also cases where tinnitus is not relieved and may even worsen after surgery.

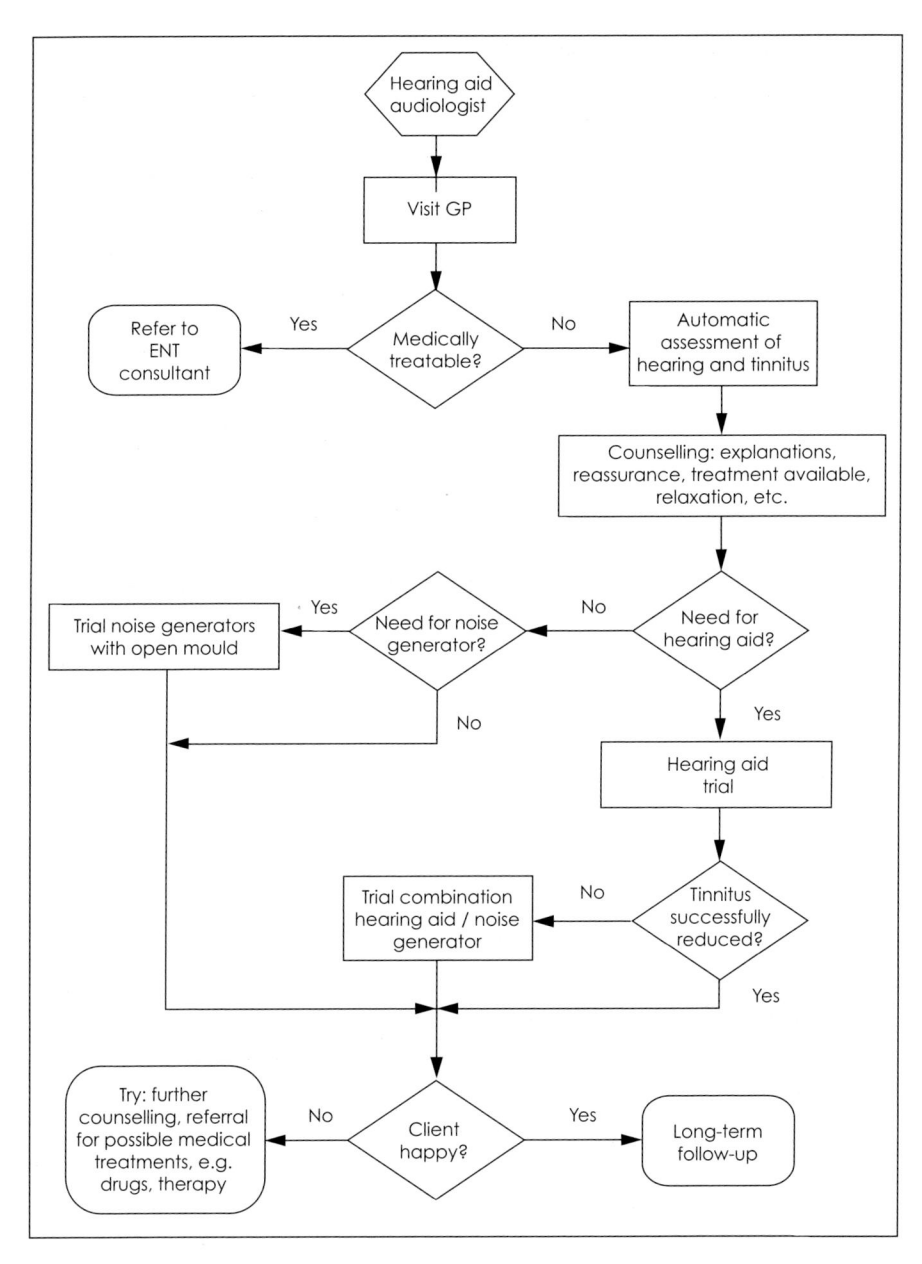

Figure 12.2 A Possible route for tinnitus sufferers

12.6.2 Alternative treatments

Where tinnitus is not amenable to medical or surgical treatment, other methods will be used which may include acoustical masking, psychotherapy, relaxation methods, physiotherapy or alternative therapies such as acupuncture or hypnotherapy. For some patients, electromagnetic stimulation (rTMS) of the brain has also been shown to be moderately helpful in temporarily inhibiting tinnitus (Langguth et al, 2008, Eichhammer et al, 2007, Landgrebe, 2008). This has been particularly successful where the tinnitus is not long-standing and the hearing is normal. Direct electrical stimulation of the auditory cortex has also been used with some effect (De Ridder, 2007).

In general, the emphasis will shift to on-going support for, whilst tinnitus is not a psychological disorder, it causes psychological problems, for example stress, tension, anxiety, poor concentration, difficulty sleeping, frustration and depression. The client is likely to need help to come to terms with the condition and to develop coping strategies.

12.6.3 Tinnitus counselling

Tinnitus counselling should be tailored to individual needs and may be directive, reactive, person-centred and/or cognitive:

- Directive counselling provides clear information about tinnitus.
- Reactive counselling responds to the client's questions.
- Person-centred counselling focuses on the needs and problems of the individual (these may not be related directly to the tinnitus) and builds on the client's strengths.
- Cognitive counselling identifies and challenges any false beliefs and attitudes or simply feelings of doom and gloom. Cognitive Behavioural Therapy (CBT) has been

shown to improve quality of life for tinnitus sufferers although it does not reduce the tinnitus itself. Cognitive counselling is usually most successful when the client has had some time 'exploring' the tinnitus with other kinds of counselling.

Tinnitus is often associated with anxiety and depression (Di Pietro et al, 2007). Counselling can help to allay the individual's fears, to overcome feelings of isolation, suggest ways to avoid trigger situations and find ways of coping with the tinnitus in everyday life. Basic counselling will usually include:

1. Explanation

   i) It is only natural to be concerned about the cause of tinnitus. It is very unlikely that the client has any serious medical condition. However it is important that they should see their general practitioner to try to find the probable cause of the tinnitus.
   ii) Tinnitus is very common and most often associated with some (possibly very slight) hearing loss. This could be due to any of a variety of causes but is often due to exposure to loud noise or simply to getting older.

2. Reassurance

   i) Tinnitus itself is a symptom and harmless.
   ii) The client should not be told that they have to learn to live with it and words like 'permanent' or 'incurable' should be avoided.
   iii) Positive statements should be used, for example that improvement is usual.

iv) Explain that tinnitus generally becomes gradually less noticeable (due to habituation – rather like traffic noise if you live for a while near a busy road).

3. Advice

Advice will generally include:

i) To avoid stress and worrying too much about the tinnitus as this can make it seem worse.
ii) Ways of 'reducing' the tinnitus for example by avoiding coffee, smoking, alcohol or other triggers and by use of low level sounds in the environment, hearing aids or masking devices to help to make the tinnitus less stark. Over time (several months) these will often improve habituation to the sound. The external sound presented is not intended to drown out the tinnitus and should be at a low level, for example just below that of the tinnitus. Quiet music is often helpful. In general, external low level sound can be helpful particularly at night when it is quiet and tinnitus is often at its most noticeable.
iii) To avoid loud noise as loud sound may increase tinnitus and many people with tinnitus also suffer from hyperacusis.
iv) Attend local individual and group tinnitus counselling.
v) Join a self-help group.

4. Support

i) Ongoing support and positive encouragement is helpful and often essential. The aim will usually be to help the client to habituate to the tinnitus so that it becomes less intrusive and no longer stressful.

ii) Fears about serious disease should be dealt with appropriately.
iii) Ongoing relaxation training and counselling may be appropriate.
iv) Where hearing aids and/or maskers are prescribed, rehabilitation with these will also be necessary.

12.6.4 Masking strategy

In quiet conditions the central auditory system increases its sensitivity so that we can detect faint sounds. This leads to an apparent increase in the loudness of all sounds – including tinnitus. Masking makes it easier for the person to filter out the sound of the tinnitus and is used to assist the habituation process.

The tinnitus assessment should indicate the likely success of a masking strategy. If there is a hearing loss, hearing aids alone may be sufficient or aids can be used in combination with maskers. Bilateral tinnitus requires bilateral masking but even unilateral tinnitus may need bilateral masking as masking one ear may result in the individual noticing tinnitus in the other ear also. The most effective masking noise is generally linked to the client's audiogram and whilst it may be the same as the tinnitus sound it is often a lower frequency. Filtered music is also used with some tinnitus patients because of its soothing effect on the regions of the brain that neuro-imaging have displayed as being the generators for the phantom perception and the distress associated with it (Sweetow, 2008). Masking or other sound therapy combined with counselling is very helpful for many clients.

Noise generators, see *Figure 12.3*, are available as:

- Non-wearable, for example under-pillow maskers.
- Instruments that look similar to hearing aids but that only produce noise.
- Combined hearing aids and noise generators.

Earmoulds used with wearable noise generators should be as open as possible because blocking the ears will heighten the tinnitus.

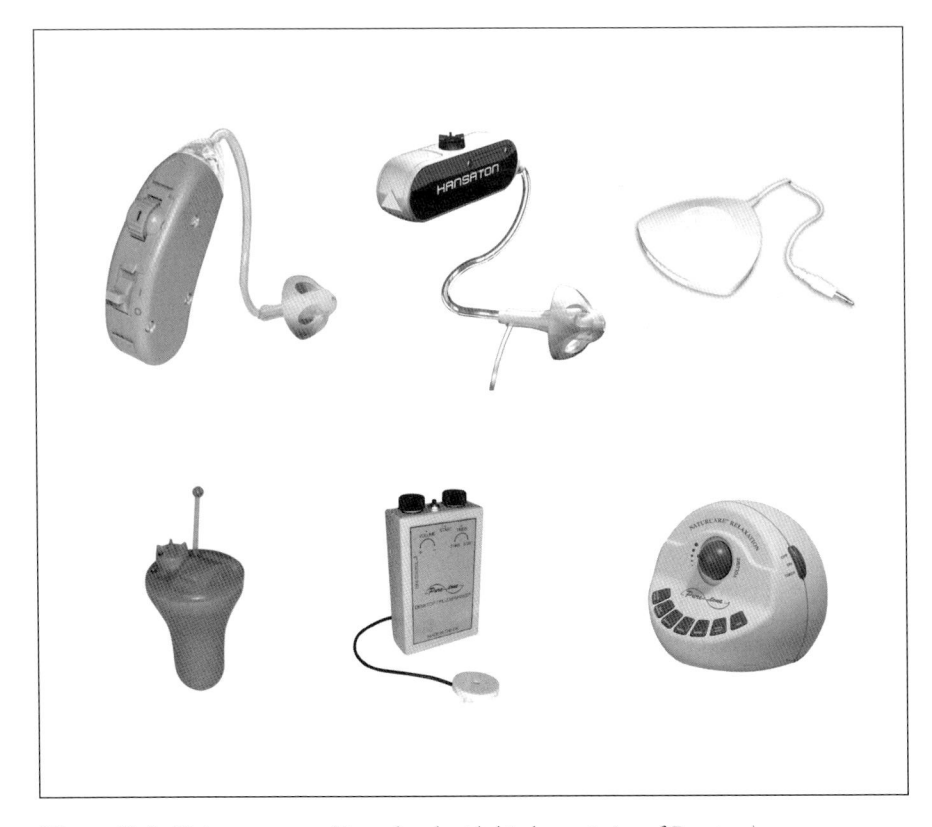

Figure 12.3 *Noise generators (Reproduced with kind permission of Puretone)*

12.6.5 Tinnitus Retraining Therapy (TRT)

Tinnitus Retraining Therapy (Jastreboff and Hazell, 1993) seeks to identify and break the cycle of stress and anxiety that either causes tinnitus or makes it worse. By so doing, the client with tinnitus can learn to cope with the problem and in many cases help relieve the severity of the symptoms. Tinnitus Retraining Therapy is a form of habituation therapy which is based on Jastreboff's neurophysiological model of tinnitus. It suggests the central nervous system is the main factor governing whether or not the tinnitus causes distress. The response of the central nervous system (CNS) in processing the abnormal signals is thought to be much more important than the loudness and other characteristics of the actual tinnitus sound. The processing may also be influenced by the client's perception of the tinnitus, for example their fear that it could be a symptom of a serious illness. The neuronal network that processes and filters the neuronal signals received by the brain is plastic, that is it is not totally fixed but can change. It is able, for example, to react to unusual sounds so that we more readily notice them. Sometimes the body responds by sweating, increased heart rate, etc. In the case of tinnitus these responses are unhelpful but they can be reduced by appropriate counselling or therapy.

TRT aims to reduce the perception of, and the distress caused by, tinnitus. It is a widely used therapy that utilises the natural process of habituation to bring lasting relief. Even where TRT is not being used, many of its concepts can be utilised by the professionals who see clients with tinnitus. The therapy includes structured counselling, sometimes over a long period of time. When their anxiety subsides, clients can learn to reduce the attention they pay to the tinnitus. This can lead to changes in the neuronal pathways and bring about a gradual habituation to the tinnitus.

Partial masking is used to speed up and enhance the habituation process. Habituation can only occur to something that is perceived, therefore completely masking out the tinnitus can delay habituation. The level of background sound used is usually just below that of the tinnitus and masking is used as much or as little as necessary but particularly during the quietest periods, including during sleep.

In general, counselling, relaxation and low level masking noise appears to be the most effective therapy. TRT provides a structured approach which utilises these features. It is sometimes only partially successful and it does not work for everyone. Intensive, prolonged and skilled counselling (whether or not TRT) is of the greatest importance in tinnitus management.

Chapter 13
Pre-Lingual Deafness

13.1 NORMAL SPEECH AND LANGUAGE DEVELOPMENT

Speech and language develops rapidly in the first few years of life. A foetus at week 30 has an almost fully developed ear and can respond to loud sounds. From birth the infant develops speech and language through well documented stages, as shown in *Table 13.1*. The infant's first three years are a period of intensive speech and language development.

Table 13.1 Stages in child speech and language development

Approximate age	Language behaviour
0-12 weeks	Reacts to loud sounds. Responds to people. Attends to speech. Moves body when listening to speech. Can differentiate between some vowel sounds. By 12 weeks can distinguish between similar consonant sounds.
3-4 months	Controls voice to make cooing sounds. Responds by turning (head and eyes) to human voices without visual cues. Responds appropriately to friendly and angry tones.

Table 13.1 Stages in child speech and language development continued

4-6 months	Babbling sounds start to emerge. Repetitive syllable production (e.g. mama). Even deaf babies start to babble. Imitates speech sounds. Uses incompletely formed plosives (b,t,d) and nasals (m,n).
6-11 months	Babbling increases. Sound play with strings of sounds (e.g. da, ma, di, du...). If the baby cannot hear babbling starts to die out. Shy with strangers. Responds to name. Points at objects. Begins to gesture to speech (e.g. wave bye bye).
12 months	Understands simple words and phrases. First words, usually nouns. Aware of social value of speech. Uses jargon (conversation-like intonational patterns). One word sentences. No longer able to distinguish sounds irrelevant to native language.
18 months	Understanding progressing rapidly. Vocabulary of up to about 50 words including nouns and verbs and other parts of speech. Can follow simple commands.
2 years	Vocabulary has grown, including nouns, verbs and other parts of speech. Two-word sentences. Able to use some common prepositions (e.g. in, on, under) also pronouns although often confuses them.

Pre-Lingual Deafness

Table 13.1 Stages in child speech and language development continued

3 years	Vocabulary has grown to 900 words including nouns, verbs, pronouns and adjectives. Basic grammar is complete. Able to use past and is developing use of future. About 90% of the child's speech is intelligible.
4 years	Vocabulary is now at about 1500 words. The essentials of language have usually been mastered. Can apply simple reason.
5+ years	Uses language in thought. Speech production and perception skills continue to increase throughout childhood. By 5, can say /m/, /p/, /b/, /h/, /w/, /k/, /g/, /t/, /d/, /n/, /ng/, /y/. By 6, can say /f/, /v/, /sh/, /th/, /l/. By 7, can say /s/, /z/, /r/, voiceless /th/, /ch/, /w/, /j/. Vocabulary increases throughout life, but at a much slower rate.

Babies start to hear before they are born. Pregnancy is divided into three trimesters. The ear is formed in the first trimester and it is most at risk during the first trimester whilst being formed. By the second trimester there is much less chance of damage. By the end of the second trimester the foetus can hear sounds from its mother's body (especially her heartbeat and stomach noises) and from the outside world. Male voices (being lower frequency) penetrate the abdomen wall better than female voices and therefore the foetus is likely to hear its father's voice better than its mother's. Loud noises can startle the foetus and cause it to make rapid leg and arm movements. Music can also stimulate or soothe it and by 32 weeks the foetus can recognise a piece of music and move in time to it! At birth the baby's hearing is much better developed than its sight.

Newborn babies (neonates) can hear well. Hearing is very important to social development and from birth they can localise sounds and turn to or from them. They start to recognise sounds in the environment, especially a parent's voice. The pitch and level is important initially and the baby is likely to be soothed by a quiet pleasant voice and to cry if they hear angry shouting. Neonates are most sensitive to loud sounds and do not respond to very quiet sounds, such as whispering. However they can discriminate between sounds that differ in intensity, frequency, duration and/or direction. Even a neonate recognises the speech features and rhythms of its parents and an English baby will prefer to look at an English speaker, whereas, for example a German baby will prefer to look at a German speaker.

Parents respond to the baby's utterances so that conversational skills such as turn-taking begin to develop. Parental (or caregiver) participation results in imitation by about six months. If a child cannot hear they will still initially develop babbling but then it starts to die out rather than developing through imitation.

The infant's first three years, see *Figure 13.1*, are a period of intensive speech and language development. Research evidence suggests that there are critical periods for speech and language development when the brain is best equipped to absorb language. Exposure to language during these periods is vital for normal development.

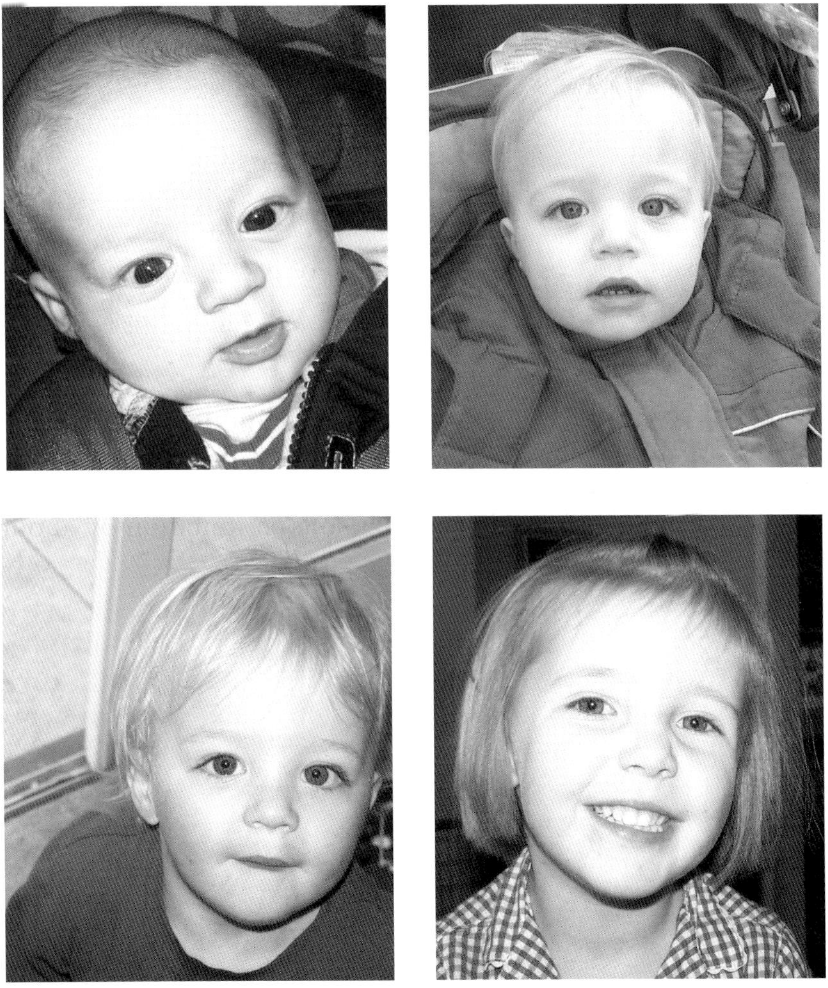

Pre-Lingual Deafness

Figure 13.1 The infant's first three years

13.2 EFFECTS OF DEAFNESS ON CHILD DEVELOPMENT

The linguist, Noam Chomsky, hypothesised that all children go through a critical learning period in their first three years during which they have an active Language Acquisition Device or LAD. Although there is considerable evidence of critical learning periods, it is still debatable how much of our language skill is innate (nature) and how much is learned (nurture).

The onset of deafness from birth or in the early years can severely disrupt the development of speech and language. Detection of hearing loss, (see *Figure 13.2*), at as early a stage as possible and the use of hearing aids is therefore vitally important to the child's progress in speech, language and education. Even minimal hearing loss can be significant for a child who is in education or is developing language. The later in life a child becomes deaf the less their speech and language will be affected. Any child who is at a disadvantage because of hearing loss should be considered for hearing aids. Spoken communication for severely and profoundly deaf children will remain slow and involve great effort on the part of both child and parents even with hearing aids fitted and educational support. The term 'parent' is used in this chapter to refer to the child's main caregiver, that is whoever is responsible for the child's care.

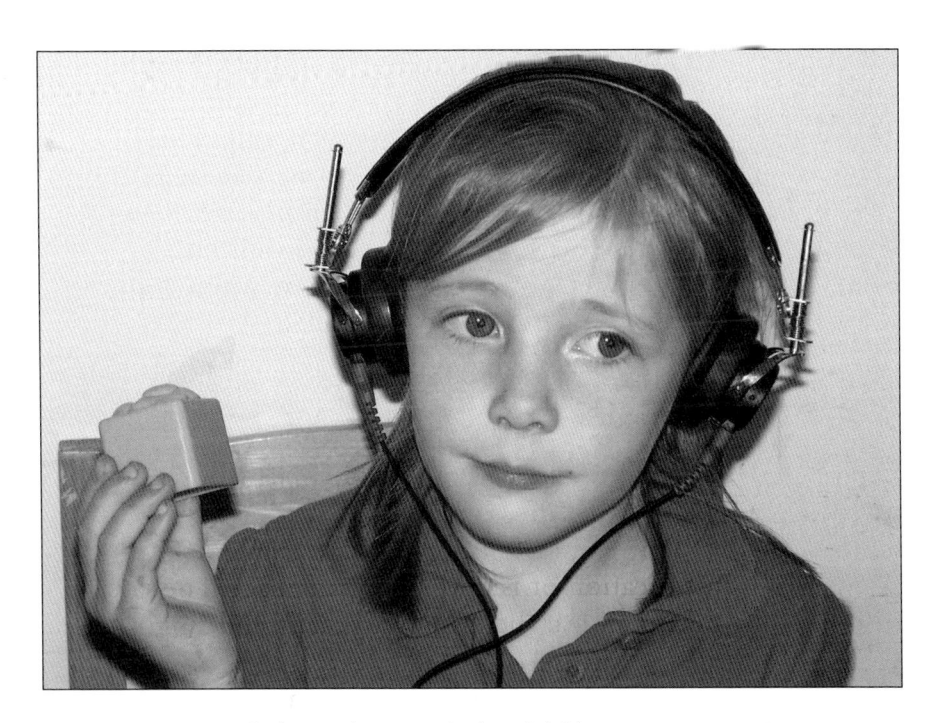

Figure 13.2 Testing for hearing loss in a school aged child

Children who are born deaf or become deaf pre-lingually (before the acquisition of language) have not yet acquired the phonemes (sounds), vocabulary and grammar of the language. They do not have a language to which they can be rehabilitated. 'Habilitation' is therefore a more appropriate term to use when talking about deaf children than 'rehabilitation'.

Early interactions between the parent and the infant are vitally important to social and emotional development. When a deaf child is born to hearing parents their interaction is likely to be impaired, regardless of the method of communication the parents choose to use. Hearing parents also tend to grieve for the 'normal' baby they never had and often feel inadequate to the task of bringing up their deaf child. For these reasons, on-going parent counselling is an important part of the deaf child's habilitation.

A deaf child born to deaf parents is much more likely to demonstrate normal patterns of social, cognitive and linguistic development because both parent and child can share the same communication system but it is important to realise that only about 3% of deaf children are born into families where both parents are deaf.

13.3 COMMUNICATION MODES

Children with lesser degrees of hearing impairment and without significant additional handicaps will invariably learn to communicate in the normal way, although their speech and language may be delayed. Parents of children who are severely or profoundly deaf will not necessarily choose for their child to use speech as their first language.

Language is central to all children's development but language should not be confused with speech. Communication with deaf children may be through speech or manual communication (sign). Manual communication can fulfil all the essential roles of spoken language but may differ in that:

- Social contact is sequential rather than simultaneous (touching and speech can occur together with spoken language).
- Visual perception develops more highly, and listening skills and sequential memory develop less well.

The choice of communication modes will be made from:

i) Auditory-oral: Spoken English is learned through listening and lipreading, supported by reading and writing.

Amplification of the child's residual hearing is key and it is important to fit hearing aids as early as possible so that sound forms part of experience, development and learning. The approach is most successful when the child is identified and aided early, whether through hearing aids or cochlear implants, and when the parents are counselled to assist and enhance their natural parenting role. Spoken language enables direct communication with the hearing world and a wide range of options in terms of education, careers and social life and the parents naturally know and are skilled at the language to be used. Nevertheless, an auditory-oral method is not an easy option. It is heavily dependent on parental involvement; success is generally slow and not all children will be successful.

ii) Cued speech uses hand shapes to indicate sounds which are not visible through lipreading alone. Cued speech is not a language in its own right as is British Sign Language. It is an oral approach that focuses on normal speech production. It is not restrictive and any word can be cued including those for which there are no signed equivalents.

iii) British Sign Language (BSL) is a manual form of communication and is visual rather than auditory. BSL is a language in its own right with its own grammar (including word order) and does not conform to spoken English. Manual communication is easier for deaf children to learn but the deaf signing community is relatively small and most hearing parents are not fluent in sign, particularly during the child's infancy, when learning language is easiest.

iv) Signed English/ Sign Supported English/ Manually Coded English consists of signs from British Sign Language (BSL) but used with English grammar, including word endings and verb tenses.

This has an obvious advantage over BSL in school in that the grammar is the same as that needed for reading and writing. However, it is not the language of the Deaf community.
v) Bilingualism is the use of Deaf sign language as the first language with English taught as a second language. This gives children access to the Deaf community and its culture whilst recognising that a fluent knowledge of English is vital for learning to read and write.
vi) Total Communication (TC) combines manual, oral and written methods of communication. The idea of TC is to use every available way to ensure the message is understood without having to choose one mode over the other. However, visual and auditory modes are very different and TC usually ends up as a compromise between the two modes (Wilcox, 1989).

Choice of the communication mode to use is usually the most difficult decision that parents have to make. The difficulty of choosing is compounded by deep disagreements between professionals about the communication options. There are significant practical, moral and emotional arguments for and against the use of each option and it is very difficult for a parent to obtain a dispassionate, unbiased view. This is particularly difficult for them as they have to make a choice early, at a stage when they are likely to be at their most vulnerable and least able to understand the full implications of the choice they are making (whichever it may be). In addition, although parents have a right to information about all the options, it does not follow that all will be available locally. Some education authorities have a specific policy that limits realistic choice.

13.4 THE EDUCATION OF DEAF CHILDREN
13.4.1 Pre-school years

About one in every thousand children is born deaf and it is estimated that about 840 children are born every year in the United Kingdom (UK) with significant (moderate to profound) deafness (National Deaf Children's Society, 2008). Overall in the UK, there are about 20,000 children aged 0-15 years who are moderately to profoundly deaf, about 12,000 of whom were born deaf.

Most parents have little or no prior knowledge of deafness and may need to access help and support. However it is important that parents retain control of the process. In the pre-school years therefore, counselling is usually provided for the parents, rather than direct education to the child. It is the professional's job to provide resources, support and information so that parents gain in the confidence and competence that will enable them to optimise their child's progress. Most parents want to collaborate with the professional to obtain the best outcomes for their child. In order for this to be achieved, the professional must respect the parents and their wishes and allow them the freedom to do things in their own way and to make their own decisions.

Most parents need specific information, skills and knowledge in order that they can optimise their deaf child's development. They need to know for example about:

- Hearing loss, its causes and effects
- Speech and language development
- Hearing aids and assistive devices
- Local support services available.

Many parents feel overwhelmed when they realise that their child will have a hearing loss for life and the feeling can be heightened by the very services intended to help the child and their family, see *Figure 13.3*. This is often particularly true due to the multiplicity of services that are involved (health, social, educational) and the differing advice that can be offered. Problems that can arise include giving too little information, giving too much information, providing information that cannot be understood by the parents, focusing only on the medical diagnosis and technical solutions, making decisions for the parents, giving the parents unrealistic tasks and generally making the parents feel guilty and inadequate.

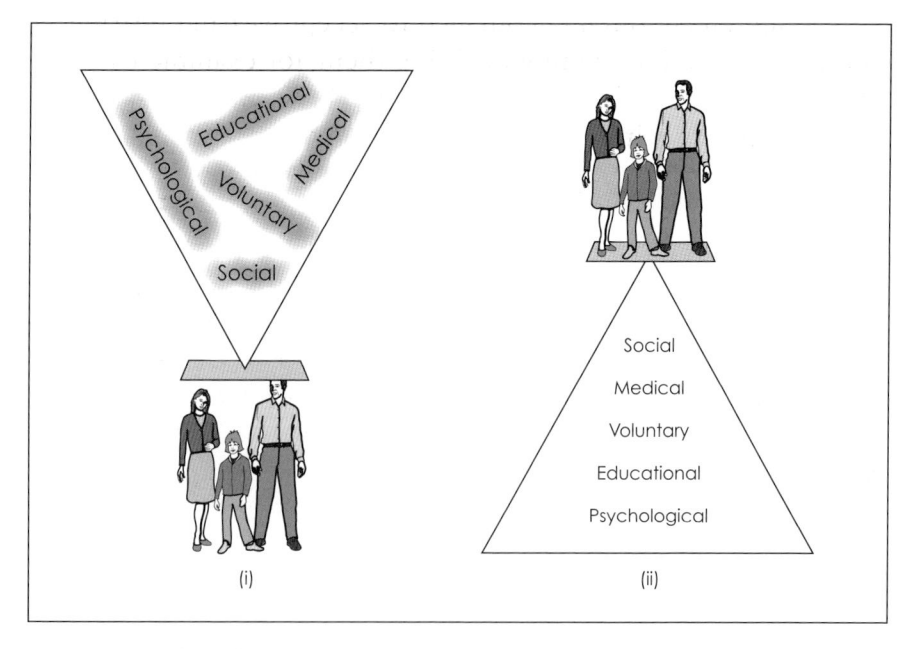

Figure 13.3 *The multiplicity of services may bear down upon the parents rather than supporting them*

The diagnosis of severe or profound hearing loss can be followed by complex emotional reactions from the parents, for example anger, guilt, denial. Professional counselling can facilitate a process of adjustment and support the family so that they can face the challenges with confidence and optimism. Expectations have to be rebuilt whilst avoiding false hopes and help should be tailored to the individual family. Many parents also find that help and support from other parents of deaf children, for sharing experiences and feelings, can be very positive.

The early fitting of appropriate amplification is vitally important for maintaining or developing aural-oral communication. Amplification should be appropriate, reliable and undistorted. It should achieve consistent (full-time) audibility for the child.

Children are often encouraged to accept wearing hearing aids and earmoulds by individualising them, for example by having them in bright colours. Radio (FM) hearing aid systems are routinely used in most school settings to overcome background noise and unfavourable classroom acoustics. Many parents also use FM whilst talking to their deaf toddlers. Audiologists who are experienced in working with deaf children will be aware of the special hearing aid needs of small children, such as using mini elbows see *Figure 13.4*, reduced sound output (because the sound is amplified in the small space available in the child's ear), compatibility with FM systems, etc. Hearing aids for children are usually dispensed through the National Health System and are therefore free of charge.

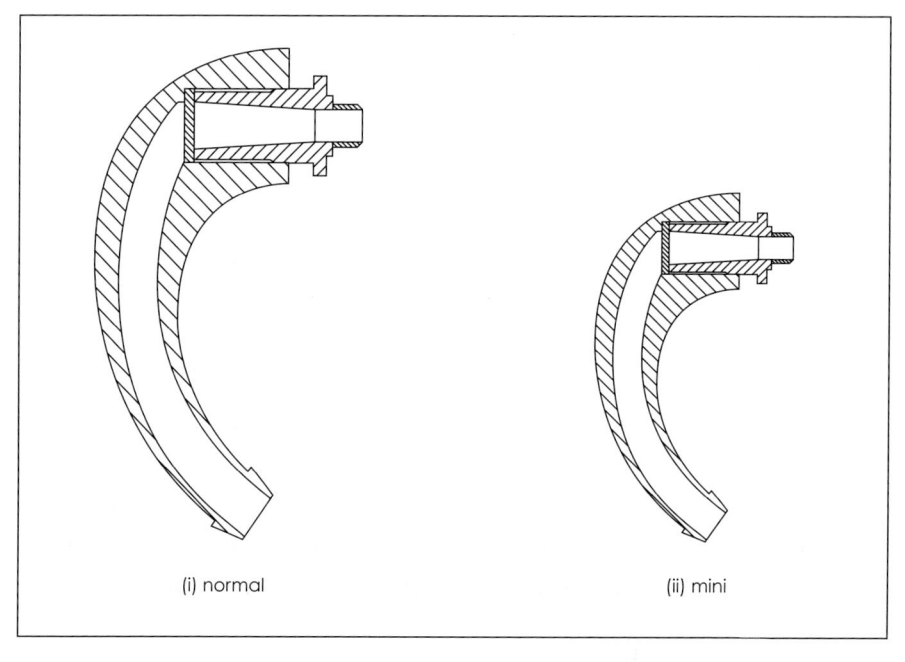

Figure 13.4 *Mini elbows*

13.4.2 School years

During the school years, specialist support is usually provided for the child and/or for the child's teacher, as most children with hearing impairment are educated in mainstream schools. Although placement in a mainstream school is relatively easy, effective inclusion of the deaf child educationally, socially, emotionally, linguistically and culturally is far from easy. The overall responsibility for meeting the child's special needs rests with the school. The type and level of educational support given varies considerably and generally depends upon factors such as:

- The child's present age
- Degree and type of deafness

- Age at onset of deafness
- Length of time without appropriate hearing aids
- Additional disabilities
- Parental involvement.

Support might, for example, involve a teacher of the deaf working with mainstream staff and providing individual structured sessions for the child, or a learning support assistant providing support within the classroom. The in-class support assistant is an adult who helps to facilitate access to the curriculum for the deaf child. There is no method of support that is without its problems, for example, the teacher of the deaf will have a case load which restricts the time that can be spent with each child, whereas the support assistant could lack adequate training and experience or might be over-supportive so that the deaf child does not develop independent learning skills.

Some schools provide a specialist resource base or 'unit' for deaf children where one or more teachers of the deaf are usually employed. A teacher of the deaf is a teacher who has undertaken additional specialised training for this role. In England and Wales a teacher working with deaf children must achieve the specialist qualification within three years.

A unit may provide a class base and main teaching area for the deaf children in the school or provide tutoring on a group and individual basis. A unit can provide the benefits of specialist knowledge and teaching, a peer group of other deaf children and supported integration. A unit is part of mainstream provision and deaf children should move between the unit and the mainstream and be included as full members of the mainstream school.

Key factors in educational success for deaf children are not so much the approach used but the quality and consistency of:

- The educational approach,
- The audiological management.

A relatively small number of severely and profoundly deaf children, and deaf children with additional disabilities, are educated in special schools. Special schools provide a highly specialised environment that offers small classes, specialised teaching and a deaf peer group. The school may be day or residential but, for many children, a special school will inevitably mean a residential setting, away from home and family.

13.5 COCHLEAR IMPLANTS

In some children the hair cells of the cochlea are lost or so badly damaged that a hearing aid is of little or no use, as no matter how much sound reaches the cochlea it cannot be transmitted to the auditory nerve and therefore no useful signals reach the brain. A cochlear implant bypasses the damaged hair cells of the cochlea and directly stimulates the auditory nerve.

Children with acquired deafness are generally very successful candidates for implantation because they already possess speech and language. Pre-lingually severely and profoundly deaf children may also be considered for cochlear implants, particularly if they are below the age of seven. If implanted early, the child may follow normal (though probably delayed) speech and language development. However, deaf parents of deaf children may not be positive towards the idea of implantation because they may view this as destructive of their Deaf culture.

Referral to a cochlear implant centre is usually via the family doctor. Referral does not commit a family but a cochlear implant team assessment can provide very valuable information, including a review of hearing aid provision and the suitability or otherwise of cochlear implants. In addition to a full case history, there will normally be an assessment of hearing, hearing aid benefit and speech and language, and a scan of the inner ear to ensure that the auditory nerve is adequate and that the formation of the cochlea will allow the electrode array to be inserted.

Cochlear implants are highly specialised hearing aids and do not restore normal hearing. Many parents believe the implants will fully restore hearing and that the child will instantly be able to understand spoken language and to talk. Cochlear implants usually lead to great positive benefits such as developing speech and language and improved confidence but they will not change a profoundly deaf child into a child with normal hearing. The implantation programme always involves extensive habilitation, usually with the main aim of achieving successful spoken communication.

Having a cochlear implant is an enormous commitment for the family. Although the cost of the implant is normally covered by the National Health Service in the United Kingdom, parents still have to find the time and expenses for numerous hospital visits. The parents have to make an informed decision about implantation. They need to understand the risks, benefits and limitations of having the device and the commitment required to the programme including the extensive post-surgery rehabilitation. Potential risks include those relating to general anaesthetic, infection, device failure and facial nerve damage. Statistically problems are uncommon but of course this is no consolation to the family if their child is the one affected. It is a difficult choice for parents to make and if the choice turns out to have been the wrong one, the parents are likely to experience guilt for having made it. Some parents write a letter to the child for the future, to explain the decision they came to, whether it was to have the implant or not:

*'Explain your state of mind, the information you have, why you
have made your decision and how you feel towards your child. Keep
it somewhere safe so that you have a record of exactly what you were
thinking at that time. If, at any time in the future, your child wants to
discuss the course you chose to take, you will have an honest account of
it, however it turned out'* (Edwards and Tyszkiewicz, 1999).

Rehabilitation after surgery is a long process, without which the child or adult will not gain full benefit. Habilitation is the process by which the child and family adapt to the hearing loss, learn how to use the implant and develop new language skills. The sounds the child hears are not the same as those heard with normal hearing and the child has to learn to interpret the new sounds.

The implant has to be maintained in good working order throughout life and this will involve on-going visits to the hospital for assessment and equipment maintenance.

13.6 CONCLUSION

Audiologists who come into contact with deaf children should provide information that is appropriate to the level of hearing loss. The family situation should be considered especially when discussing education and mode of communication. Parents are likely to be overwhelmed and professionals must work together if they are to support the parents rather than adding further confusion, helplessness and frustration. Professionals should give practical advice and straightforward information to guide the parents as they explore the options and reach their own decisions. Audiologists who work with young children are usually specially trained to do so, as this is a critical time in the habilitation process and parental support is crucial.

Appendix

252   Adult Aural Rehabilitation

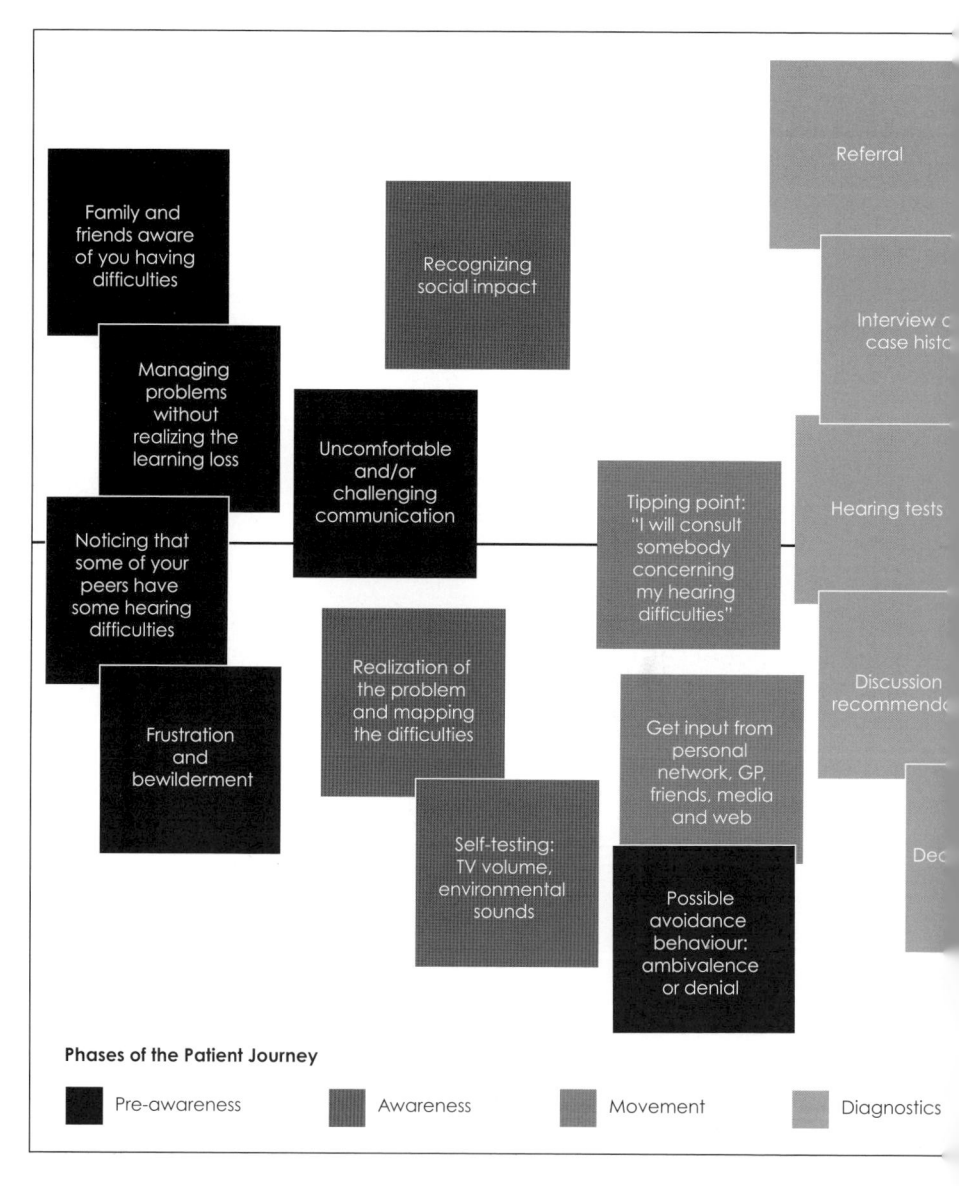

Phases of the Patient Journey

- Pre-awareness
- Awareness
- Movement
- Diagnostics

Pre-awareness phase:
- Family and friends aware of you having difficulties
- Managing problems without realizing the learning loss
- Noticing that some of your peers have some hearing difficulties
- Frustration and bewilderment
- Uncomfortable and/or challenging communication
- Possible avoidance behaviour: ambivalence or denial

Awareness phase:
- Recognizing social impact
- Realization of the problem and mapping the difficulties
- Self-testing: TV volume, environmental sounds

Movement phase:
- Tipping point: "I will consult somebody concerning my hearing difficulties"
- Get input from personal network, GP, friends, media and web

Diagnostics phase:
- Referral
- Interview c case histo
- Hearing tests
- Discussion recommendc
- Dec

The 'Possible Patient Journey' shown here is a tool that can be altered by the audiologist to reflect each individual patient's experience (Kindly supplied by the Ida Institute www.idainstitute.dk)

Appendix

- Social impact
- Counselling
- Ongoing self-evaluation
- Hearing solutions
- Assistive technology
- Adaptation and change
- Problems satisfactorily resolved (or not resolved)
- Treatment
- Communication strategies
- Identification of new problems
- Accept or reject treatment

Rehabilitation   Post-clinical

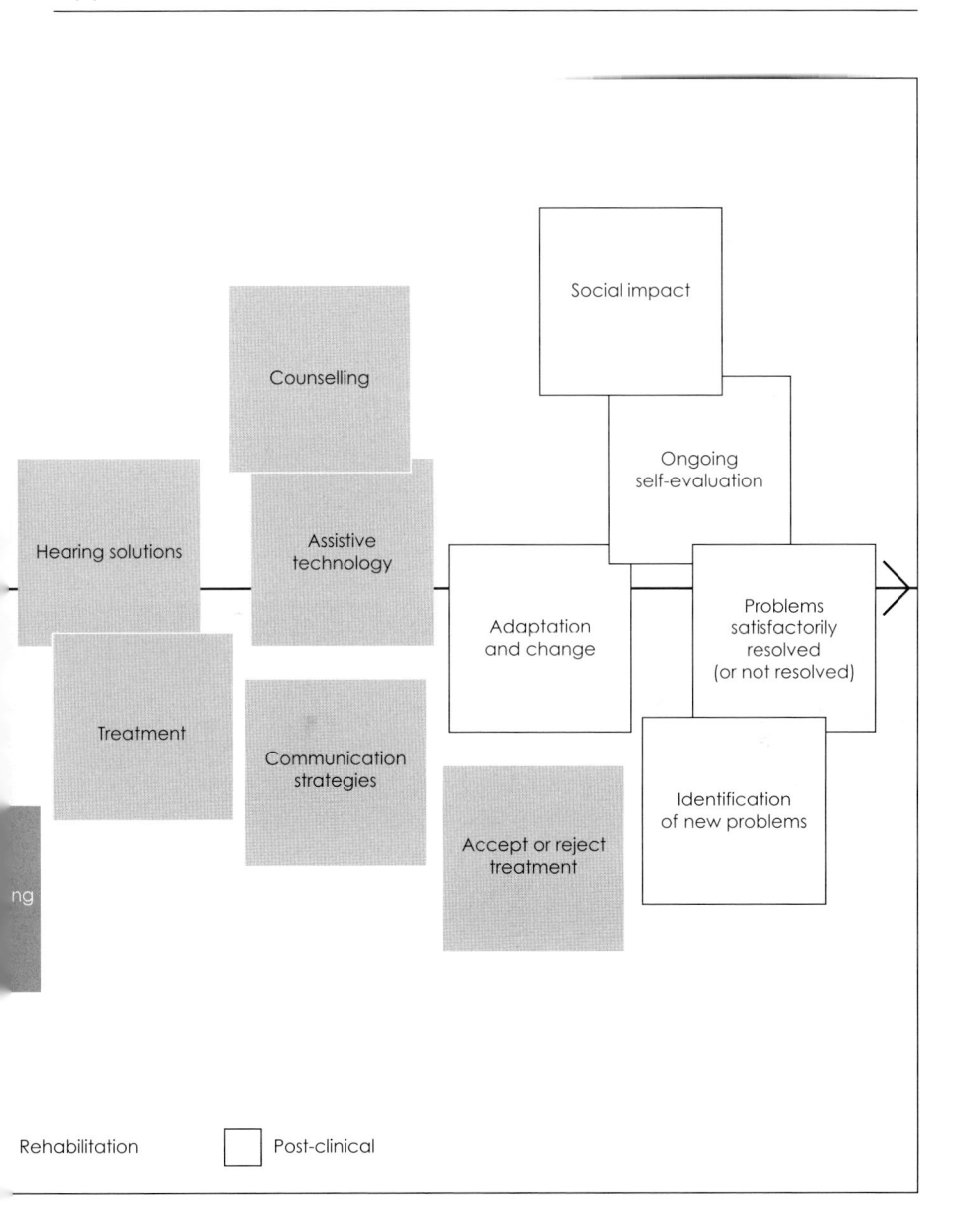

Bibliography

Alpiner, J.G. & McCarthy, P.A. (1993). *Rehabilitative Audiology. Children and Adults.* 2nd edition. Philadelphia: Lippincott Williams and Wilkins.

Aviv, A. & Harley, C.B. (2001). How long should telomeres be? *Current Hypertension Reports.* 3, pp.145–151.

Barsky, A.J. (1981). Hidden reasons some patients visit doctors. *Annals of Internal Medicine.* 94, pp.492-498.

Bateson, G. (1972). *Steps to an Ecology of Mind: Collected Essays in Anthropology, Psychiatry, Evolution, and Epistemology.* Chicago: University Of Chicago Press.

Bentler, R.A. and Kramer, S.E. (2000). Guidelines for choosing a self-report outcome measure. *Ear and Hearing.* 21, 37S-49S.

Bernstein Lewis, C. (2002). *Aging: The Health Care Challenge.* 4th edition. Philadelphia: F.A. Davis.

Birren, J.E. & Schaie, K.W. eds., (2005). *Handbook of the Psychology of Aging. 5E (Handbooks of Aging).* 6th edition. New York: Academic Press.

Blake, R. & Sekuler, R., (2006). *Perception.* 5th edition. Columbus, OH: McGraw Hill.

Bodner, A.G. Ouellette, M. Frolkis, M. Holt, S.E. Chiu, C.P. Morin, G.B. Harley, C.B. Shay, J.W. Licheseiner, S. Wright, W.E. (1998). Extension of life-span by introduction of telomerase into normal human cells. *Science.* 279, pp.349–352.

Braisby, N. and Gellatly, A., (2005). *Cognitive Psychology.* Oxford: Oxford University Press in association with The Open University.

Brody, D.S. & Miller, S.M., (1986). Illness concerns and recovery from a URI. *Medical Care.,* 24, pp.742-748.

Brody, D.S. Miller, S.M. Lerman, C.E. Smith, D.G. & Caputto, G.C., (1989). Patient perception of involvement in medical care: relationship to illness attitudes and outcomes. *Journal of General Internal Medicine.* 4, pp.506-511.

Brooks, D.N., ed., (1989). *Adult Aural Rehabilitation.* London: Chapman and Hall.

Carlson, N.R., (2001). *Psychology of Behaviour.* 7th edition. Needham Heights, MA: Allyn and Bacon.

Clark, J.G. & Martin, F.N., eds., (1994). *Effective Counselling in Audiology. Perspectives and Practice.* Upper Saddle River, NJ: Prentice Hall.

Coren, S. Ward, L.M. & Enns, J.T., (2003). *Sensation and Perception.* 5th edition. Orlando, FL: Harcourt College Publishers.

Corker, M., (1994). *Counselling – The Deaf Challenge.* London: Jessica Kingsley Publishers.

Cox, R.M., (1996). The Abbreviated Profile of Hearing Aid Benefit (APHAB) - Administration and application. *Phonak Focus.* No. 21.

Cox, R.M., (1997). Administration and application of the APHAB. *Hearing Journal.*, 50(4), pp.32-48.

Cox, R.M., (2003). Assessment of subjective outcome of hearing aid fitting: getting the client's point of view. *International Journal of Audiology.*, 42, pp.S90-S96.

Cox, R. & Alexander, G., (2007). Personality, hearing problems, and amplification characteristics: contributions to self-report hearing aid outcomes. *Ear and Hearing.*, 28(2), pp.141-162.

Cox, R.M. & Alexander, G.C., (1995). The Abbreviated Profile of Hearing Aid Benefit (APHAB). *Ear and Hearing.*, 16(2), pp.176- 186.

Cox, R.M. & Alexander, G.C., (1992). Maturation of hearing aid benefit: objective and subjective measurements. *Ear and Hearing.*, 13, pp.131-141.

Cox, R.M. & Gilmore, C., (1990). Development of the Profile of Hearing Aid Performance (PHAP). *Journal of Speech and Hearing Research.* 33, pp.343-357.

Cox, R.M. Gilmore, C.G. & Alexander, G.C., (1991). Comparison of two questionnaires for patient-assessed hearing aid benefit. *Journal of the American Academy of Audiology.*, 2, pp.134-145.

Cox, R.M. & Rivera, I.M., (1992). Predictability and reliability of hearing aid benefit measured using the PHAB. *Journal of the American Academy of Audiology.*, 3, pp.242-254.

Crowe, T., ed., (1997). *Applications of Counselling in Speech-Language Pathology and Audiology.* Baltimore: Williams and Wilkins.

Davis, A., (1995). *Hearing in Adults.* London: Whurr.

De Jong, P.J., (2002). Implicit self-esteem and social anxiety: differential self-favouring effects in high and low anxious individuals. *Behaviour Research and Therapy.* 40(5), pp.501-508.

Devlieger, P. Rusch, F. & Pfeiffer, D., eds., (2003). *Rethinking Disability: The Emergence of New Definitions, Concepts and Communities.* Leuven/Apeldoorn: Garant Publishers.

Effros, R. B., (2005). Roy Walford and the immunologic theory of aging. *Immunity and Ageing.,* 2, p.7.

Egbert, L.D. Batitt, G.E. Welch, C.E. & Bartlett, M.K., (1964). Reduction in postoperative pain by encouragement and instruction of patients. *New England Journal of Medicine.* 270, pp.825-827.

Eisenthal, S. & Lazare, A., (1976). Evaluation of the initial interview in a walk-in clinic. *Journal of Nervous and Mental Disease.,* 162, pp.169-176.

Erber, N.P., (1985). *Telephone Communication and Hearing Impairment.* London: Taylor and Francis.

Falvo, D.R., (2005). *Medical and Psychosocial Aspects of Chronic Illness and Disability.* 3rd ed. Sudbury: Jones and Bartlett Publishers.

Field, A. P., (2006). Is conditioning a useful framework for understanding the development and treatment of phobias? *Clinical Psychology Review.*, 26(7), pp.857-875.

Gagne, J.P. Stelmacovich, P. & Youetich, W., (1991). Reactions to requests for clarification used by hearing impaired individuals. *Volta Review.*, 93, pp.129-143.

Gagne, J.P. & Wyllie, A., (1989). Relative effectiveness of three repair strategies on the visual identification of misperceived words. *Ear & Hearing.* 10(6), pp.368-74.

Goffmen, E., (1963). *Stigma: Notes on the Management of Spoiled Identity.* London: Penguin.

Goldsmith, T., (2004). Aging as an evolved characteristic – Weismann's theory reconsidered. *Medical Hypotheses.*, 62(2), pp.304-308.

Goldstein, D.R. & Stevens, S.D.G., (1981). Audiological rehabilitation: management model 1. *Audiology.*, 20, pp.432-52.

Hall, J.A. Roter, D.L. & Katz, N.R., (1988). Correlates of provider behaviour: a meta-analysis. *Medical Care.* 26, pp.657-675.

Harley, C.B. Vaziri, H. Counter, C.M. Allsopp, R.C., (1992). The telomere hypothesis of cellular aging. *Experimental Gerontology.*, 27, pp.375–382.

Harman, D., (1956). Aging: a theory based on free radical and radiation chemistry. *Journal of Gerontology.* 11(3), pp.298-300.

Harman, D., (1972). A biologic clock: the mitochondria? *Journal of the American Geriatrics Society.*, 20(4), pp.145-147.

Harper, P.S. (1994). The epidemiology of Huntington's disease. *Human Genetics.* 89,4, 365-376.

Harper, P. S. Quarrell, O. W.J Youngman, S. Hodgson, S.V. McLaren, A L. Cassiman, J.-J., (1988). Huntington's disease: prediction and prevention (and discussion). *Philosophical Transactions of the Royal Society of London Series B, Biological Sciences* (1934-1990). 319(1194), pp.285-298.

Headache Study Group of the University of Western Ontario (1986) Predictors of outcome in headache patients presenting to family physicians – a one-year prospective study. *Headache Journal.* 26, 285-294.

Hersen, M. & Van Hasselt,V.B., eds., (1998). *Handbook of Clinical Gerontology.* New York: Springer.

Hogan, A., (2001). *Hearing Rehabilitation for Deafened Adults. A psychosocial approach.* London: Whurr.

Holliday, R., (2002). Twenty years of ageing research at the Mill Hill Laboratories. *Experimental Gerontology.*, 37(7), pp.851-857.

Hosford-Dunn, H. & Halpern, J., (2000). Clinical application of the Satisfaction with Amplification in Daily Life Scale in private practice 1: statistical, content, and factorial validity. *Journal of the American Academy of Audiology.*, 11, pp.523-539.

Hull, R.H., (1997). *Aural Rehabilitation. Serving Children and Adults.* 3rd edition. San Diego, CA: Singular Publishing Group.

Jasper, M., (2003). *Beginning Reflective Practice – Foundations in Nursing and Health Care.* Cheltenham: Nelson Thornes.

Johnson, C E & Danhauer, J.L., (2002). *Handbook of outcomes measurement in Audiology.* Albany, NY: Delmar Learning.

Jung, C.G., (1933). *Modern man in Search of a Soul.* San Diego, CA: Harcourt, Brace and World Inc.

Kaplan, S.H. Greenfield, S. & Ware, J.E., (1989). Assessing the effects of physician–patient interactions on the outcomes of chronic disease. *Medical Care.,* 27(3), pp.S110-127.

Kenworthy, O.T., (1986). Caregiver-child interaction and language acquisition of hearing impaired children. *Topics in Language Disorders,.* 6(3), pp.123-133.

Kim, S. Kaminker, P. & Campisi, J., (2002). Telomeres, aging and cancer: In search of a happy ending. *Oncogene.,* 21, pp.503-511.

Kleinman, A. Eisenberg, L. & Good, B., (1978). Culture, illness and care: clinical lessons from anthropologic and cross-cultural research. *Annals of Internal Medicine.,* 88, pp.251-258.

Kochkin, S., (1996). Customer satisfaction and subjective benefit with high performance hearing aids. *The Hearing Review.,* 3(12), pp.16-26.

Korsch, B.M. Gozzi, E.K. & Francis, V., (1968). Gaps in doctor–patient communication. *Pediatrics.,* 42, pp.855-871.

Korzybski, A., (1994). *Science and Sanity: An Introduction to Non-Aristotelian Systems and General Semantics.* 5th Edition. Fort Worth, TX: Institute of General Semantics.

Langguth, B. Hajak, G. Kleinjung T. Cacace, A. & Moller, A.R. (2007). *Tinnitus: Pathology and Treatment. Progress in Brain Research.,* Vol. 166. Amsterdam: Elsevier.

Lars, R. & Bergman, R.B., (2000). *Developmental Science and the Holistic Approach.* New Jersey: Lawrence Elbaum Associates.

Lilienfeld, S.O. Lynn, S.J. & Lohr, J.M., eds., (2004). *Science and Pseudoscience in Clinical Psychology.* New York: Guilford Press.

Luxon, L., ed., (2003). *Textbook of Audiological Medicine. Clinical Aspects of Hearing and Balance.* London: Martin Dunitz.

Marschark, M., (1993). *Psychological development of Deaf Children.* Oxford: Oxford University Press.

Neurotone, (2008). LACE 3.0 *Auditory Training Manual for Hearing Health Care Professionals.* Redwood City, CA: Neorotone Inc.

Newell, A. & Simon, H. A., (1972). *Human Problem Solving.* Upper Saddle River, NJ: Prentice Hall.

Newman, C.W. Weinstein, B. E. Jacobson, G. P. & Hug, G. A. (1990). The Hearing Handicap Inventory for Adults: psychometric adequacy and audiometric correlates. Amplification and aural rehabilitation. *Ear & Hearing.* 11(6), pp.430-433.

Oliveira, C.A., (2007). How does stapes surgery influence severe disabling tinnitus in otosclerosis patients? *Advanced Otolaryngology.,* 65, pp.343-347.

Orth, J.E. Stiles, W.B. Scherwitz, L. Hennrikus, D. & Vallbona, C., (1987). Patient exposition and provider explanation in routine interviews and hypertensive patients' blood pressure control. *Health Psychology.,* 6, pp.29-42.

Paul, R.G. & Cox, R.M., (1995). Measuring hearing aid benefit with the APHAB: Is this as good as it gets? *American Journal of Audiology.,* 4(3), pp.10-13.

Pervin, L. A., ed., (1990). *Handbook of Personality: Theory and Research.* New York: Guilford Press.

Philosophical Transactions of the Royal Society of London, (1988). The Prevention and Avoidance of Genetic Disease. Series B. *Biological Sciences.,* Vol. 319(1194), pp. 285-298.

Plomp, R., (1978). Auditory handicap of hearing impairment and the limited benefit of hearing aids. *Journal of Speech and Hearing Research.,* 29, pp.146-154.

Rogers, C.R., (1951). *Client-centred Therapy.* Boston, MA: Houghton Mifflin.

Rosenfeld, R.H. & Wilson, D.C., (1999). *Managing organisations.* 2nd edition. New York: McGraw-Hill.

Roter, D.L., (1977). Patient participation in the patient-provider interaction. The effects of patient question asking on the quality of interaction, satisfaction and compliance. *Health Education Monographs.,* 5(4), pp.281-15.

Roter, D.L. Hall, J.A. & Kern, D.E. Barker, L.R. Cole, K.A. & Roca, R.P., (1995). Improving physicians interviewing skills and reducing patients emotional distress. *Archives of Internal Medicine.* 155, pp.1877-1884.

Sala, S., ed., (1999). *Mind Myths: Exploring Popular Assumptions About the Mind and Brain.* Chichester: John Wiley and Sons.

Schow, R., (2001). A standardized AR battery for dispensers is proposed. *The Hearing Journal.,* 54(8), pp.10-20.

Schow, R.L. & Nerbonne, M.A., (2007). *Introduction to Audiologic Rehabilitation.* 5th edition. Needham Heights, MA: Allyn and Bacon .

Silverman, J. Kurtz, S. & Draper, J., (1998). *Skills for communicating with patients.* Oxford: Radcliffe Press.

Singer, J.L., ed., (1990). *Repression and Dissociation. Implications for Personality Theory, Psychopathology, and Health.* Chicago: The University of Chicago Press.

Stephens, D., (2002). Audiological Rehabilitation. In: Luxon, L. Furmans, J.M. Martini, A. & Stephens, D., eds. *Textbook of Audiological Medicine. Clinical Aspects of Hearing and Balance.* London: Martin Dunitz. Ch. 30.

Sweetow, R.W. & Henderson Sabes, J., (2006). The Need for and Development of an Adaptive Listening and Communication Enhancement (LACE) Program. *Journal of the American Academy of Audiology.*, 17(8), 538-558.

Tuckett, D.A. Bouton, M. & Olson, C., (1985). A new approach to the measurement of patients' understanding of what they are told in medical consultations. *Journal of Health and Social Behaviour.* 26, pp.27-38.

Tyler, R.S., ed., (2000). *Tinnitus Handbook.* San Diego, CA: Singular Press.

Waitzkin, H., (1985). Information giving in medical care. *Journal of Health and Social Behavior.*, 26(2), pp.81-101.

Walford, RL., (1969). *The Immunologic Theory of Aging.* Copenhagen: Munksgaard.

Weiner, I.B. Freedheim, D.K. Gallagher, M. Schinka, J.A. & Velicer, W.F., (2003). *Handbook of Psychology.* Chichester: John Wiley & Sons.

Weinstein, B.E., (2000). *Geriatric Audiology.* New York: Thieme.

Weismann, A. Poulton, E.B. Schonland, S. & Shipley, A.E., (1891). (Digitised 2007). *Essays upon heredity and kindred biological problems.* Oxford: Clarendon Press.

Williams, G. C., (1957). Pleiotropy, natural selection and the evolution of senescence. *Evolution.*, 11, pp.398-411.

References

Adams, J.D. Hayes, J. & Hopson, B., (1977). *Transition: Understanding and Managing Personal Change.* Oxford: Wiley-Blackwell.

Aitchison, J., (2000). *The Seeds of Speech: Language Origin and Evolution.* Cambridge: Cambridge University Press.

Allen, R.E. ed., (1991). *The Concise Oxford Dictionary.* 8th edition. London: Book Club Association.

American Psychiatric Association, (1994). *Diagnostic Statistical Manual of Mental Disorder (DSMIV).* 4th edition. Arlington, VA: American Psychiatric Association.

Atchley, R.C., (1974) The meaning of retirement. *Journal of Communication.*, 24, pp.97-101.

Atchley, R.C., (2000). *Social Forces and Aging.* 9th edition. Belmont, CA: Wadsworth.

Atchley, R.C., (2006). The meaning of retirement. *Journal of Communication.*, 24(4), pp.97-100.

Aubert, G. & Lansdorp, P. M., (2008). Telomeres and aging. *Physiological Reviews.* 88, pp.557-579.

Bandler, R. & Grinder, J., (1979). *Frogs into Princes: Neuro linguistic Programming.* Moab, UT: Real People Press.

Bandler, R., Andreas, S. & Andreas, C. eds., (1985). *Using Your Brain-for a Change.* Indian Hills, CO: NLP Comprehensive.

Bartels, H. Staal, M.J. & Albers, F., (2007). Tinnitus and neural plasticity of the brain. *Otology and Neurology.,* 28(2), pp.178-184.

Bayne, S. & Liu, J.P., (2005). Hormones and growth factors regulate telomerase activity in ageing and cancer. *Molecular and Cellular Endocrinology.* 240(1-2), pp.11-22.

Beck, A.T., (1972). *Depression: Causes and Treatment.* Philadelphia, PA: University of Pennsylvania Press.

Beck, A.T., (1985). *Anxiety, Disorders and Phobias.* New York: Basic Books.

Beck, J.S., (1995). *Cognitive therapy: Basics and beyond.* New York: Guilford.

Betts, D.H. & Madan, P., (2008). Permanent embryo arrest: molecular and cellular concepts. *Molecular Human Reproduction.,* 14, pp.445-453.

Bienfield, D. ed., (1990). *Clinical Geropsychiatry.* 3rd edition. Baltimore: Williams and Wilkins.

Birren, J.E. & Fisher, L.M., (1995). Aging and speed of behavior: possible consequences for psychological functioning. *Annual Review of Psychology.,* 46, pp.329-353.

Blood, I.M. & Blood, G.W., (1999). Effects of acknowledging a hearing loss on social interactions. *Journal of Communication Disorders.*, 32(2), pp.19-120.

Bodnar, A.G. Ouellette, M. Frolkis, M. Holt, S.E. Chiu, C. Morin, G.B. Harley, C.B. Shay, J.W. Lichtsteiner, S. & Wright, W.E., (1998). Extension of life-span by introduction of telomerase into normal human cells. *Science.*, 279(5349), pp. 349 – 352.

Botswick, J.M. & Pankratz, V.S., (2000). Affective disorders and suicide risk: a reexamination. *American Journal of Psychiatry.*, 157, pp.1925-1932.

Collins, C.R. & Blood, G.W., (1990). Acknowledgement and severity of stuttering as factors influencing nonstutterers' perceptions of stutterers. *Journal of Speech and Hearing Disorder.*, 55, pp.75-8.

Cox, R.M. & Alexander, G.C., (1995). The Abbreviated Profile of Hearing Aid Benefit (APHAB). *Ear and Hearing.*, 16(2), pp.176- 186.

Cox, RM & Gilmore, C., (1990). Development of the Profile of Hearing Aid Performance (PHAP). *Journal of Speech and Hearing Research.*, 33, pp.343-357.

Davis, A., (1995). *Hearing in Adults.* London: Whurr.

Davis, C ,(1990). Psychosocial Aspects of Aging. In Lewis, C.B., ed. *Aging: The Health Care Challenge.* 2nd edition. Philadelphia.

De Filippo, C.L., (1988). Tracking for speechreading training. *Volta Review.*, 90, pp.215-239.

Demeester, K. Van Wieringen, A. Hendick, J. Tropsakal, V. Fransen, E. Van Laer, L. Van Camp, G & Van de Hayning, P., (2009) Audiometric shape and presbyacusis. *International Journal of Audiology.* 48, 4, 222-232.

De Ridder, D. De Mulder, G. Menovsky, T. Sunaert, S & Kovacs, S., (2007) Electrical Stimulation of auditory and somatosensory cortices for treatment of timitus and pain. *Prog Brain Res.,* 166, pp 377-88.

Di Clemente, C.C. Prochaska, J.O. Fairhurst, S.K. Velicer, W.F. Velasquez, M.M. & Rossi, J.S., (1991). The process of smoking cessation: An analysis of precontemplation, contemplation and preparation stages of change. *Journal of Consulting and Clinical Psychology.* 59, pp.295-304.

Dillon, H. James, A. & Ginis, J., (1997). The Client Oriented Scale of Improvement (COSI) and its relationship to several other measures of benefit and satisfaction provided by hearing aids. *Journal of the American Academy of Audiology.,* 43, pp.85-99.

Dilts, R.B. & De Lozier, J.A., (2000). *Encyclopedia of Systemic Neuro-Linguistic Programming and NLP New Coding.* Scotts Valley, CA: NLP University Press.

Di Pietro, G. Carrabba, L. Giannini, P. Marciano, E. Speranza, B. Cerruti, C. Petrosino, M. Nardo, M.P. & Valoroso, L., (2007). Evaluation of the psychopathological risk factors associated with tinnitus: A case-control study of an outpatient cohort. *Audiological Medicine.,* 5(2), pp.125-128.

Dobson, K.S., ed., (2001). *Handbook of Cognitive –Behavioural Therapies.* 2nd edition. New York: Guilford Press.

Eichhammer, P. Kleinjung, T. Landgrebe, M. Hajak, G. & Langguth, B., (2007). *TMS for treatment of chronic tinnitus: neurobiological effects*. In Langguth, B. Hajak, G.,

Edwards, J. & Tyszkiewicz, E., (1999). Cochlear Implants. In J.Stokes, ed. *Hearing Impaired Infants. Support in the First Eighteen Months.* London: Whurr. Ch. 6.

Engel, G.L., (1977). The need for a new medical model: A challenge for biomedicine. *Science.* 196(4286), pp.129–36.

Epel, E.S. Blackburn, E.H. Lin, J. Dhabhar, F.S. Adler, N.E. Morrow, J.D. & Cawthon, R.M., (2004). Accelerated telomere shortening in response to life stress. *Proceedings of the National Academy of Sciences.,* 101(49), pp.17312-17315.

Erber, N.P., (1996). *Communication Therapy for Adults with Sensory Loss.* 2nd edition. Clifton Hill, Victoria, Australia: Clavis Publishing.

Erber, N.P., (2002). *Hearing, Vision, Communication and Older People.* Clifton Hill, Victoria, Australia: Clavis Publishing.

Erber, N.P., (2003). Use of hearing aids by older people; influence of non-auditory factors (vision, manual dexterity). *International Journal of Audiology.,* 42(2S), pp.21-25.

Eysenck, H.J., (1967). *The Biological Basis of Personality.* New York: Thomas.

Field, A.P., (2000). *The Psychology of Attitudes.* Orlando, FL: Harcourt Brace. Jovanovich College Publishers.

Freud, S., (1926). Publication of Inhibitions, Symptoms and Anxiety and The Question of Lay Analysis. Cited in J. L. Singer, (1995). *Repression and Dissociation: Implications for Personality Theory, Psychopathology, and Health.* Chicago: University of Chicago Press.

Garfield, B., (2006). Cited in R. Atkinson 'I hoped our baby would be deaf'. *The Guardian.*, March 21st.

Gatehouse, S., (1997). The Glasgow hearing aid benefit profile: A client-centred scale for the assessment of auditory disability, handicap and hearing aid benefit. Poster presented at *The American Academy of Audiology.*, Fort Lauderdale.

Gatehouse, S., (1999). Glasgow Hearing Aid Benefit Profile: Derivation and validation of a client-centered outcome measure for hearing aid services. *Journal of the American Academy of Audiology.*, 10, pp.80-103.

Ghaye, T. Cutherbert, S. Danai, K. & Dennis, D., (1996). *Learning through Critical Reflective Practice. Self Supported Learning Experiences for Health Care Professionals.* Newcastle upon Tyne: Tyne Pentaxion Ltd.

Gibbs, G.,(1988). *Learning by Doing: A Guide to Teaching and Learning Methods.* Oxford: Further Education Unit, Oxford Brookes University.

Gilley, D. Tanaka, H. & Herbert, B.S., (2005). Telomere dysfunction in aging and cancer. *International Journal of Biochemical Cell Biology.*, 37 (95), pp.1000-13.

Giolas, T.G. Owens, E. Lamb, S.H. & Schubert, E.D., (1979). The Hearing Performance Inventory (HPI). *Journal of Speech and Hearing Disorders.*, 44, pp.169-195.

Goldsmith, T. C., (2004). Aging as an evolved characteristic – Weismann's theory reconsidered. *Medical Hypotheses.*, 62 (2), pp. 304-308.

Hajak, G. Langguth, B. Landgrebe, M. Nyuyki, K. Frank, E. Steffans, T. Hauser, S. & Eichhammer, P., (2008). Effects of colour exposure on auditory and somatosensory perception – hints for cross-modal plasticity. *Neuro Endocrinology Letters.*, 29, p.4.

Haldane, J. B. S., (1941). *New Paths in Genetics.* London: George Allen & Unwin Ltd.

Harley, C.B. Vaziri, H. Counter, C.M. & Allsopp, R.C., (1992). The telomere hypothesis of cellular aging. *Experimental Gerontology.*, 27, pp.375–382.

Harman, D., (1956). Aging: a theory based on free radical and radiation chemistry. *Journal of Gerontology.*, 11(3), pp.298-300.

Haussmann, M. F. & Mauck, R. A., (2008). Telomeres and longevity: testing an evolutionary hypothesis. *Molecular Biology and Evolution.* 25, pp.220-228.

Hayflick, L., (1965). The limited in vitro lifetime of human diploid cell strains. *Experimental Cell Research.*, 37, pp.614–636.

Hayflick, L., (1996). *How and Why we Age.* New York; Ballantine Books.

Hawkins, D., (1990). Technology and hearing aids: How does the audiologist fit in? *Journal of Speech, Language and Hearing Research.*, 32, pp.42-43.

Hawkridge, A., (1987). Cited in Sheppard, L. & Hawkridge, A. (1987). *Tinnitus. Learning to Live With It.* Bath: Ashgrove Press.

Hitch, G.J., (2005). Working Memory. In Braisby N. & Gellatly A., eds., *Cognitive Psychology.*, Oxford: Oxford University Press.

Humes, L.E., (1999). Dimensions of hearing aid outcome. *Journal of the American Academy of Audiology.*, 10, pp.26-39.

Ida Institute, Copenhagen, Denmark.

Jastreboff, P.J. & Hazell, J.W.P., (1993). A neurophysiological approach to tinnitus: clinical implications. *British Journal of Audiology.*, 27, pp.1-11.

Johnson, C.E. & Danhauer, J.L., (2002). *Handbook of Outcome Measurement in Audiology.* Florence, KY: Cengage Learning.

Jones, W.H.S., (1951). *Loeb Classical Library.*, Vol 6, Book 20, Section 162. Cambridge, MA: Harvard University Press.

Judson, A., (1991). *Changing Behavior in Organizations: Minimizing Resistance to Change.* Oxford: Basil Blackwell.

Jung, C. G., (1933). *Modern Man in Search of a Soul.* Orlando, FL: Harcourt, Brace & World.

Kaplan, H. Bally, S.J. & Garretson, C., (1985). *Speechreading: A Way to Improve Understanding.* Washington, DC: Gallaudet University Press.

Keay, D.G. & Murray, J.A.M., (2007). Hearing loss in the elderly : a 17-year longitudinal study. *Clinical Otolaryngology.*, 13(1) pp.31-35.

Kemp, B., (1988). Motivation, rehabilitation and aging: A conceptual model. *Topics in Geriatric Rehabilitation.*, 3(3), pp.41-52.

Kim, S-H Kaminker, P. Campisi, J., (2002). Telomeres, aging and cancer: in search of a happy ending. *Oncogene.*, 21, pp.503-511.

Kim, N.W. Piatyszek, M.A. Prowse, K.R. Harley, C.B. West, M.D. Ho, P.L. Coviello, G.M. Wright, W.E. Weinrich, S.L. Shay, J.W., (1994). Specific association of human telomerase activity with immortal cells and cancer. *Science.*, 266, pp.2011-2015.

Kirkwood, T.B.L. & Rose M.R., (1991). Evolution of senescence: late survival sacrificed for reproduction. *Philosophical Transactions: Biological Sciences.*, 332(1262), pp.15-24.

Kleinjung, T. Eichhammer, P. Landgrebe, M. S. & P. Hajak, G. Steffens, T. Strutz, J. & Langguth, B., (2008). Combined temporal and prefrontal transcranial magnetic stimulation for tinnitus treatment: a pilot study. *Otolaryngology Head Neck Surgery.* 138(4), pp.497-501.

Kochkin, S., (2002). Factors impacting customer choice of dispenser and hearing aid brand; use of ALDs & computers. *Hearing Review.*, 9(12), pp.14-23.

Kolb, D. A., (1984). Experiential Learning: *Experience as the Source of Learning and Development.* Upper Saddle River, NJ: Prentice-Hall.

Kubler-Ross, E. (2005). *On Grief and Grieving: Finding the Meaning of Grief Through the Five Stages of Loss.* New York: Simon & Schuster Ltd.

Lamb, S.H. Owens, E. & Schubert, E.D., (1983). The revised form of the Hearing Performance Inventory. *Ear and Hearing.*, 4(3), pp.152-157

Landgrebe, M. Binder, H. Koller, M. Eberl, Y. K. Leinjung, T. & Eichhammer, P., (2008). *BioMed Central Psychiatry.*, 8(1) p.23.

Lane, H., (1992). *The Mask of Benevolence: Disabling the Deaf Community.* New York: Alfred A. Knopf.

Lane, H. Hoffmeister, R. & Bahan, B., (1996). *A Journey into the Deaf-world.* San Diego, CA: Dawn Sign Press.

Lane, N. (2005). *Power, Sex, Suicide: Mitochondria and the Meaning of Life.* Oxford: Oxford University Press.

Langguth, B. Kleinjung, T. Frank, E. Landgrebe, M. S. & P. & Dvorakova, J., (2008). High-frequency priming does not enhance the effect of low-frequency rTMS in the treatment of tinnitus. *Experimental Brain Research.*, 184(4), pp.587-591.

References

Langguth, B. Kleinjung, T. Fischer, B. Hajak, G. Eichhhammmer, P. & Sand, P.G., (2007). Tinnitus severity, depression, and the big five personality traits. In Langguth, B. Hajak, G. Kleinjung, T. Cacace, A. & Moller, A.R., eds. *Progress in Brain Research., Vol. 166, Tinnitus: Pathophysiology and Treatment.* New York: Elsevier.

Lindley, G., (2006). Current hearing aid fitting protocols: results from an online survey. *Audiology Today.*, 18(3), 19-22.

Maltby, M., (2002). *Principles of Hearing Aid Audiology.* London, : Whurr.

Maltby, M., (2005). *Occupational Audiometry: Monitoring and Protecting Hearing at Work.* Oxford: Butterworth Heinemann.

Maslow, A.H., (1968). *Toward a Psychology of Being.* 2nd edition. New York: Van Nostrand Reinhold.

Medawar, P.B., (1952). *An Unsolved Problem of Biology.* Cherry Hill, NJ: H.K. Lewis.

Montgomery, A., (1994) WATCH: A practical approach to brief auditory rehabilitation. *The Hearing Journal.* 4 (10)

Montgomery, A. & Houston, W., (2000). Management of the Hearing impaired Adult. In: J. Alpiner & P. McCarthy (Eds.) *Rehabilitative Audiology: Children and Adults.* 3rd edition. Baltimore: Williams & Wilkins.

Morera, O.F. Johnson, T.P. Freels, S. Parsons, J. Crittenden, K.S. Flay, B.R. & Warnecke, R.B., (1998). The measure of stage of readiness to change: Some psychometric considerations. *Psychological Assessment.*, 10, pp.182-186.

National Deaf Children's Society, (2008). [Online]. Available at: http://www.ndcs.org.uk/for_the_media/faqs.html#faqblock4

Newman, C.W. Jacobsen, G.P. & Spitzer, J.B., (1996). Development of the Tinnitus Handicap Inventory. *Archives of Laryngology - Head Neck and Surgery.*, 122(2), pp.143-148.

Office for National Statistics, (2004). *Living in Britain. The 2002 General Household Survey.* London: Office of Population Censuses and Surveys. Ch. 11. [Online]. Available at: http://www.statistics.gov.uk/lib2002/downloads/hearing.pdf

Oliver, M. (1983). *Social work with Disabled People.* Oxford: Macmillans.

Parasnis, I., ed., (1996). *Cultural and Language Diversity and the Deaf Experience.* Cambridge: Cambridge University Press.

Paykel, E.S., (1989). The Background, Extent and Nature of the Disorder. In Herbst K. and Paykel E.S., eds. *Depression: An Integrative Approach.* Oxford: Heinemann Medical Press.

Pearl, R., (1926). *Alcohol and Longevity.* New York: Alfred A. Knopf.

Pichora-Fuller, M.K & Benguerel, A., (1991). The Design of CAST (Computer-Aided Speechreading Training). *Journal of Speech and Hearing Research.* Vol.34(1), 202-212.

Plant, G., (1996). *Commtrac: Modified Connected Discourse Tracking Exercises for Hearing Impaired Adults.* Chatswood, Australia: National Acoustic Laboratories.

Prochaska, J.O. & Di Clemente, C.C., (1983). Stages and processes of self-change of smoking: Towards an integrative model of change. *Journal of Consulting and Clinical Psychology.*, 51, pp.390-395.

Rehm, J. Ustum, T. & Saxema, S., (1990). On the development and psychometric testing of the World Health Organisation screening instrument to assess disablement in the general population. *International Journal of Methods in Psychiatric Research.*, 8, pp.110-122.

RNID (2008). [Online]. Available at: http://www.rnid.org.uk/information_resources/factsheets/deaf_awareness/factsheets_leaflets/facts_and_figures_on_deafness_and_tinnitus.htm#deafened

Rodier, F. Kim, S.H. Nijjar, T. Yaswen, P. & Campisi, J., (2005). Cancer and aging: the importance of telomeres in genome maintenance. *International Journal of Biochemistry and Cell Biology.*, 37(5), pp.977-90.

Rogers, C.R., (1951). *Client-centred Therapy.* Boston, MA: Houghton Mifflin.

Salama, R., (2008). Dementia: symptoms, diagnosis and management. *Nurse Prescribing.*, 6(8), pp.362 - 367.

Slavi, R.J. Lockwood, A & Burkard, R. (2000). Neural Plasticity and Tinnitus. In Tyler, R.S. (ed) *Tinnitus Handbook.* Singular Publishing.

Sanders, D.A., (1993). *Aural Rehabilitation. A Management Model.* 2nd edition. Upper Saddle River, NJ: Prentice Hall Inc.

Schön, D.A., (1983). *The Reflective Practitioner: How Professionals Think in Action*. London: Temple Smith.

Silverman, J. Kurtz, S. & Draper, J.,(1998). *Skills for Communicating with Patients*. Oxford: Radcliffe Press.

Sweetow, R., (2008). *Effects of musical stimulation on concentration, relaxation and tinnitus*. Unpublished talk given to the Association of Independent Hearing Healthcare Professionals (AIHHP), Cambridge 10th October.

Sweetow, R.W. & Henderson-Sabes, J., (2004). LACE: Listening and auditory communication enhancement training. *The Hearing Journal.*, 57(3), pp.32-38.

Tate, S. & Sills, M., (2004). *The development of critical reflection in the health professions*. London: Learning and Teaching Network, Centre for Health Sciences and Practice.

Tye-Murray, N., (1998). *Foundations of Aural Rehabilitation*. San Diego, CA: Singular Publishing Group Inc.

Tye-Murray, N., (2002). *Conversation Made Easy: Speechreading and Conversation Strategies Training for People With Hearing Loss*. St Louis: Central Institute for the Deaf.

Vassilopoulos, S., (2008). Coping strategies and anticipatory processing in high and low socially anxious individuals. *Journal of Anxiety Disorders.*, 22(1), pp.98-107.

Ventry, I. M. & Weinstein, B. E., (1982). The Hearing Handicap Inventory for the Elderly: a new tool. *Ear & Hearing.*, 3(3), pp.128-134.

Walden, B. Demorest, M. & Helper, E.L., (1984). Self-report approach to assessing benefit derived from amplification. *Journal of Speech and Hearing Research.*, 27, pp.49-56.

Walford, R.L., (1969). *The Immunologic Theory of Aging.* Copenhagen: Munksgaard.

Wilcox, S., (1989). *American Deaf Culture.* Burtonsville, Maryland: Linstok Press.

Williams, G.C., (1957). Pleiotropy, natural selection and the evolution of senescence. *Evolution.*, 11, pp.398-411.

Wolfersdorf, M., (1986). Depression and suicidal behaviour. Psychopathological differences between suicidal and non-suicidal depressive patients. *Archives of Suicide Research.* [Online]. Available at: http://priory.com/adsui3.htm [Accessed 15 Nov 2008].

World Health Organization, (1994). *International Classification of Impairments, Disabilities, and Handicaps: A Manual of Classification Relating to the Consequences of Disease.* Geneva: Office of Publications, World Health Organization.

World Health Organization, (2001). *International Classification of Functioning, Disability and Health (ICF).* Resolution WHA54.21. Geneva: Office of Publications, World Health Organization.

Index

Abbreviated Profile of Hearing Aid Benefit (APHAB)	186-188
Acceptance	6, 103, 104, 161
Access to work scheme	213
Acclimatisation, hearing aid	70, 87, 94-97
Acoustic feedback	89
Acquired deafness	8, 28, 82, 101
Active listening	72-73
Age group	14-16
Ageing	37-60
Ageing, social effects of	47-52
Ageing, theories of	53-60
Age-related changes	37-48
Aggressive behaviour	152
Agnosia	31
Agrammartism	31
Air conduction hearing aids	77-78
Alerting devices	197-198
Alzheimer's disease	52
Amplification	10, 22, 77-87
Analogue signal processing	82-83
Anchoring strategies	179
Anger	102-103
Anomia	31

Anxiety — 167–171
   models — 168–169
APHAB see Abbreviated Profile of Hearing Aid Benefit
Aphasia — 31
Approaches
   behavioural — 115–116, 157, 175
   biological — 175
   psychodynamic — 175
Apraxia — 31
Areas of the brain — 18–19, 30, 33–34
Assertive behaviour — 152
Assessment
   rehabilitation — 9, 61, 63–64, 66, 183–194, 211
   tinnitus — 221–223
Assistive devices — 195–213
Attitude
   client — 4–5, 160
   towards deafness — 27–28
   types — 4–5
Audiogram — 23, 47–48, 69–71, 141–142
Audiometric descriptors — 24
Audiometric tests — 49, 61, 66, 222
Auditory
   cortex — 18–19, 30, 225
   nerve — 18–19, 30
   pathways of the brain — 30
   phantom — 219
   training — 12, 121–148
Auditory-oral communication — 240–242
Autism — 31
Auto-immune theory — 55

Index

Background noise	26-27, 98, 100
Beck, Aaron	172
Behaviour	
aggressive	152
assertive	152
modification	116
passive	151
Behavioural	
approach	116-118, 157, 175
therapy	170, 175-176
Behaviourist theory	116-118
Bilateral hearing loss	26
Bilingualism	29, 241-242
Binaural hearing aids	86-87
Biological	
approach	175
clock	56-57
Bio-psychosocial model of disability	113
Bone conduction hearing aids	78
Brain	
areas of and functions	18, 32-35, 218, 220
damage	31-35
British Sign Language	16, 29, 241
Broca's aphasia	34
BSL, see British Sign Language	
Care and maintenance of hearing aids	87-93
Case history	9, 63-65
CAST, see Computer Aided Speech-reading Training	
Causes of tinnitus	218-220
Change	
process	1-2, 114-115
transition curve	103-106
Changes in touch	47

Chemical damage 54-56
Children 16-17, 20, 82, 212-213, 217, 233-250
Chomsky, Noam 238
Classification, World Health Organisation 7-8, 111-113
Cleaning of hearing aids 87, 89-92
Client
    expectations 6, 97, 104, 161, 245
    journey see Patient journey
Client Orientated Scale of Improvement (COSI) 192-193
Client-centred therapy 118-120, 149, 157
Closed questions 73-74
Cochlea 19, 23, 43-44, 218
Cochlear implants 79-82
Cognitive behavioural therapy (CBT) 176, 225-226
Cognitive
    changes 36, 48-49
    therapy 116-117, 157, 170, 174-175
Cognitive-behavioural approaches 116-117, 175-176, 225
Communication 17-18, 121, 122-126
    difficulties 1, 3, 25-26, 101, 121-122, 183
    modes 240-242
    partner, training 125-126
    problems 1, 24-25, 100-101, 121-122, 183, 238
    repair 124-125
    skills 8, 72-74, 149-154
    strategies 123-129, 162-164, 176
    training 123-124, 125-126
Comprehension, speech 17-18, 22, 24
Compression 84-85
Computer Aided Speech-reading Training (CAST) 133-134
Computer-based auditory training programmes 132-135
Conditioning, behaviour 117, 169
Conductive hearing loss 20-21, 78

Index

Consonants	22, 68-69, 130, 138-141, 142
perception of	22, 138-139
Consumer model	155
Continuous discourse tracking	131-132
'Conversation Made Easy'	134-135
Conversational style	122-123
COSI see Client Orientated Scale of Improvement	
Counselling	114-120, 149-165
approaches	157
consumer model	155
definition	149
expert model	155, 156
informational	149-150, 159-160
principles	152
problem identification	158-159
referral	164-165
skills	149-150, 153-154
tinnitus	27, 225, 230, 231
transplant model	155
Criterion referencing	185
Critical learning periods	238
Cued speech communication	241
Cues	40, 72, 74, 143, 153
Cultural model of disability	114
Data logging, hearing aid	97
Deaf	
community	28-29, 112, 114-115, 242
culture	114
Deafness	
acquired	82, 101
attitudes towards	27-28
in children	233-250
post-lingual	25

pre-lingual	25, 233-250
Dementia	52
Demonstration hearing aids	70
Denial	2, 102, 104
Depression	103, 171-176
Desensitisation	170
Digital	
hearing aids	82-83
signal processing	80, 82-86
Direct audio input (DAI)	199, 210, 211
Directional microphone	83-84, 86
Disability	7-8, 111-114
Disabled Students' Allowance	213
Dysarthria	32
Dysfluency	32
Dysphonia	32
Dyspraxia	31
Ear development during pregnancy	235
Earmould	
care	91-92
fitting	89, 92-93
modifications	88
retubing	93
Education	4-6, 174, 212-213, 243-248
of deaf children	243-248
services	212-213, 243
Employment	100, 213
Endocrine theory	55
Environmental factors	38, 45
Evaluation	
measures	183-194
rehabilitation	62, 183-195, 211-212

Index

Evolutionary theories	56–59
Existential therapy	119
Expectations	104, 161, 165, 244
Expert model	155–156
Feedback	
acoustic	70, 89
auditory	130, 148
control systems	83, 86
FM radio aids see Frequency modulated (FM) radio aids	
Free field speech tests	70
Free radical theory	55
Frequency modulated (FM) radio aids	210–211, 245
Freudian theory	115–116
Gender differences	14–15
Genetic	
factors	38, 43, 53, 55
theories	56–59
Gerontology	53
Gestalt approach	120
GHABP see Glasgow Hearing Aid Benefit Profile	
Glasgow Hearing Aid Benefit Profile (GHABP)	188–191
Goal setting	161, 174
Grief	102–103
Group training	126–129
Guilt	101, 245, 249
Habilitation	8
Habituation therapy	230
Handicap	7–8
HAPI see Hearing Aid Performance Inventory	

Hearing aid
    acclimatisation   **70, 87, 94-97**
    cleaning   **87, 89-92**
    data logging   **97**
    feedback   **70, 89**
    feedback control systems   **83, 86**
    management   **87-94**
    programmes   **86**
    purpose   **77**
    types   **69, 77-78**
Hearing Aid Performance Inventory (HAPI)   **191-192**
Hearing aids   **13, 77-98**
    air conduction   **77-78**
    binaural   **86-87**
    bone conduction   **78**
    care and maintenance   **87-93**
    digital   **82-83**
Hearing Handicap Inventory for the Elderly (HHIE)   **191**
Hearing loss
    bilateral   **26**
    conductive   **20-21, 78**
    effect of   **1-4, 26**
    mild   **24**
    mixed   **19**
    moderate   **24**
    profound   **13, 16, 24, 29, 148, 245, 248**
    sensorineural   **21-23, 43, 45**
    severe   **24**
    speed of onset of   **25-26**
    sudden onset of   **26, 148**
    unilateral   **26-27**
Hearing Performance Inventory (HPI)   **193-194**

Index

Hearing	
tactics	**12, 98, 145**
test	**66–69**
HHIE see Hearing Handicap Inventory for the Elderly	
Hiatus hernia	**53**
Hormonal changes	**40, 55, 59**
HPI see Hearing Performance Inventory	
HPI-R see Hearing Performance Inventory	
Huntingdon's disease	**53, 58**
Hyperacusis	**216, 217, 227**
Hyperexcitability syndrome	**218**
Induction loop	**200, 201, 204–208, 210**
Informational counselling	**149–150, 159–160**
Infra red systems	**209**
Initial consultation	**63–65**
Intelligence	**49**
Kolb learning cycle	**74–76**
LACE, see Listening and Communication Enhancement	
Language Acquisition Device (LAD)	**238**
Lipreading	**142–143, 162–163**
Listening and Communication Enhancement	**132–133**
Localisation of sound	**26, 86**
Long term average speech spectrum	**141**
Loop systems	**200, 201, 204–208, 210**
portable	**200, 201, 208**
Maladaptive strategies	**121–122**
Manual communication	**28, 240–241, 242**
Masking strategy, tinnitus	**228–229**
Maslow's hierarchy of need	**108**
Medical model of disability	**109**

Memory	**47-48**
activities	**131, 133**
Microphones, directional	**83-84, 86**
Mild hearing loss	**24**
Misphonia	**217**
Models of	
anxiety	**168-169**
disability,	
bio-psychosocial	**113**
cultural model	**114**
medical	**111**
social	**111-114**
Moderate hearing loss	**24**
Modes of communication	**240-242**
Modifications, earmould	**88**
Motivation	**160-161**
Musculo-skeletal changes	**40-41**
Mutation accumulation theory	**58-59**
National Health Service	**212, 249**
Neural activity, tinnitus	**218-220**
Neurolinguistic programming (NLP)	**176-181**
Neurolinguistics	**31**
NHS see National Health Service	
NLP see Neurolinguistic programming	
Noise generators	**229**
Noise reduction systems	**86**
Non-verbal cues	**72, 153**
Norm referencing	**186**
Old age	**37-53**
Open questions	**73-74**
Osteoperosis	**52**

Parkinson's disease	52-53
Passive behaviour	151
Pathology of tinnitus	218-220
Patient journey	
Perception, speech	34, 139-141
Phonemes	139, 140, 141
Phonophobia	217
Place theory	218-219
Plaques and tangles	52
Population studies	13-17
Portable loop systems	200, 201, 208
Post-lingual deafness	25
Pregnancy, ear development during	235
Pre-lingual deafness	25, 114, 233-250
Presbyacusis	42, 45-46
Presbyopia	47
Problem solving	115-116, 162-164
strategies	114-115, 118-119, 162-164
Profound hearing loss	13, 16, 24, 29, 148, 245, 248
Programmed theory	54, 56-57
Psychoanalytic approaches	115-116
Psychodynamic	
approach	175
therapy	171
Psychotherapy	115-116
Public attitudes to deafness	27-28
Questioning techniques	73-74
Questionnaires	61, 184-194
Questions	
closed	73-74
open	73-74

Radio aids 210-211, 245
Reaction time 49
Recruitment 22-23, 216, 217
Referral for further counselling 164-165
Reflective practice 74-76
Reframing strategies 179-180
Rehabilitation
    assessment 9, 61, 63-64
    definition 8
    evaluation 185-194
    process 9-12, 61-63, 107
    on-going 62, 97, 107
Rejection 3-4, 100-101
Reliability theory 55
Repair strategies, communication 124-125, 163-164
Retirement 50-51
Retrocochlear damage 23-24
Retubing earmoulds 93
Role changes 51, 101

Self-assessment measures 185-194
Sensory changes 42-43
Severe hearing loss 24
SHAPI 192
Sight difficulty 11, 46-47, 60
Sign language 16, 28-29, 110, 241
Signal processing
    analogue 82-83
    digital 80, 82-86
Signal-to-noise ratio 195
Signed English 241
Significant other 101, 161
Social
    effects of ageing 25, 50-51

model of disability	111-113
services	212
Speech and language	
development	233-237, 243, 248
disorders	30-31, 34-35
Speech	
chain	17-18
comprehension	69
perception	34, 139-141
production	135-139, 148, 233-236
reading	98, 126, 142-144
recognition activities	131
sounds	135-142
spectrum, long term average	141
tests, free field	70
tracking	131-132
Speed of onset of hearing loss	25-26
Stages of rehabilitation	61-63, 102-107, 114-115, 180
Statistics	13-17
Stigma	2-3, 28
Strategies	
anchoring	179
reframing	179-180
Stress	150-152
Sudden onset of hearing loss	25-26, 148
Support services	212-213
Tactics, hearing	12, 98, 145
Teacher of the deaf	247
Telecoil	204-208, 210
Telephone	
assistive devices	197, 198, 201-202, 203
training	144-147
text	201-202

Telomeres	**56-57**
Theories of Ageing	**53-60**
auto-immune	**55**
endocrine	**55-56**
free radical	**55**
genetic	**56-59**
mutation accumulation	**58-59**
programmed	**56**
rate of living	**54**
reliability	**55**
wear and tear	**54-56**
Therapy	
behavioural	**170, 175-176**
cognitive	**115-116, 157, 170, 174-175**
psychodynamic	**171**
tinnitus retraining (TRT)	**27, 230-231**
Tinnitus	**13, 27, 215-231**
counselling	**27, 225-228, 230, 231**
handicap assessment	**221-223**
Handicap Inventory	**222**
management	**223-231**
masking strategy	**228-229**
Retraining Therapy (TRT)	**27, 230-231**
treatments	**218, 220, 223, 225**
causes	**218-220**
medical referral	**220**
neural activity	**220**
pathology of	**218-220**
triggers	**219-220, 226, 227**
Total communication (TC)	**242**
Transplant model	**155**
Unilateral hearing loss	**26-27**

Index

VAT and assistive devices	212
Verbal cues	72, 141-142, 153-154
Vision	11, 46-47, 60
Visual changes	46-47
Vocal tract	135, 136, 137
Voluntary organisations	213
Vowel recognition	136-137
Wax traps	90-91
WDRC see Wide dynamic range compression	
Wear and tear theories	54-56
Wernicke's area	18, 34
WHO classifications see World Health Organisation classifications	
WHO, see World Health Organisation	
Wide dynamic range compression (WDRC)	84-85
Wireless Systems	204-211
World Health Organisation (WHO)	7-8
classifications	7-8, 112, 113